Anatomy & Physiology

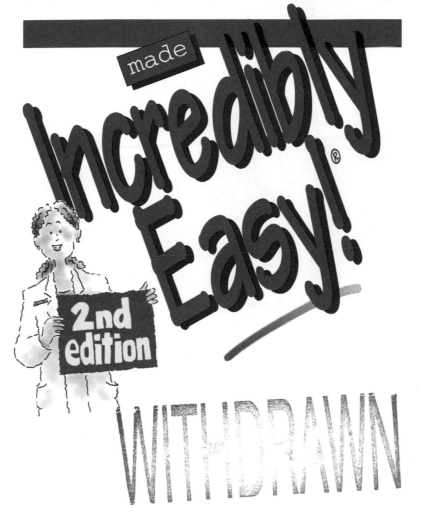

made **Incredibly Easy!**®

2nd edition

WITHDRAWN

Anatomy & Physiology

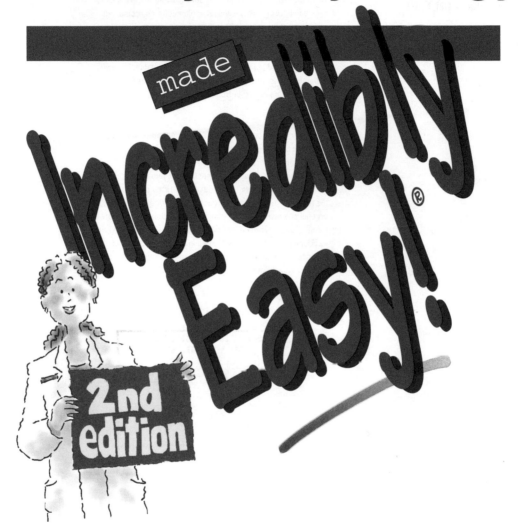

made Incredibly Easy!®

2nd edition

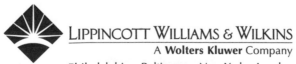

LIPPINCOTT WILLIAMS & WILKINS
A **Wolters Kluwer** Company

Philadelphia • Baltimore • New York • London
Buenos Aires • Hong Kong • Sydney • Tokyo

Staff

Executive Publisher
Judith A. Schilling McCann, RN, MSN

Editorial Director
David Moreau

Clinical Director
Joan M. Robinson, RN, MSN

Senior Art Director
Arlene Putterman

Art Director
Mary Ludwicki

Editorial Project Manager
Jaime Stockslager Buss

Clinical Project Manager
Jana L. Sciarra, RN, MSN, CRNP

Editors
Laura Bruck, Jo Donofrio, Julie Munden,
Gale Thompson

Clinical Editors
Maryann Foley, RN, BSN;
Anita Lockhart, RN, C, MSN

Copy Editors
Kimberly Bilotta (supervisor), Amy Furman,
Lisa Stockslager, Pamela Wingrod

Designers
Lynn Foulk, Donna Morris

Illustrators
Bot Roda

Digital Composition Services
Diane Paluba (manager), Joyce Rossi Biletz,
Richard Eng

Manufacturing
Patricia K. Dorshaw (director), Beth Janae Orr

Editorial Assistants
Megan L. Aldinger, Tara L. Carter-Bell,
Linda K. Ruhf

Indexer
Barbara Hodgson

APMIE2E—D
06 05 04   10 9 8 7 6 5 4 3 2

Library of Congress Cataloging-in-Publication Data

Anatomy & physiology made incredibly easy. — 2nd ed.
    p. ; cm.
    Includes bibliographical references and index.
    1. Human physiology — Outlines, syllabi, etc. 2. Human anatomy — Outlines, syllabi, etc. I. Title: Anatomy and physiology made incredibly easy. II. Lippincott Williams & Wilkins.
    [DNLM: 1. Anatomy. 2. Physiological Processes. QS 4 A5385 2005] QP41.A53 2005

612 — dc22
ISBN 1-58255-301-7 (alk. paper)   2004000460

Contents

Contributors and consultants

Gary J. Arnold, MD
Associate Professor
College of Nursing & Allied Health
 Professions
University of Louisiana at Lafayette

Edna Atwater, RN
Administrative Director
Duke University Medical Center
Durham, N.C.

Peggy Bozarth, RN, MSN
Professor of Nursing
Hopkinsville (Ky.) Community College

Karen A. Brown, MS, MT(ASCP), CLS
Associate Professor and MLT Program
 Director
University of Utah Department of
 Pathology
Salt Lake City

Marsha L. Conroy, RN, BA, MSN, APN
Nurse Educator
Cuyahoga Community College
Cleveland
Kent (Ohio) State University

Anneliese Dudley-Seals, RN, MSN
Nursing Instructor
Lamar State College
Port Arthur, Tex.

**Patricia (Pady) Dunn, RN, MSN, CNCCC,
 CNephC**
Clinical Associate Professor
University of British Columbia
Vancouver

Christian C. Evans, PhD, MSPT, ACSM
Assistant Professor, Physical Therapy
 Program
Midwestern University
Downers Grove, Ill.

Michelle L. Foley, RN,C, MA
Director of Nursing Education
Charles E. Gregory School of Nursing
Raritan Bay Medical Center
Perth Amboy, N.J.

Sherry W. Fox, RN, PhD, CNRN
Assistant Professor of Nursing
University of Virginia
Charlottesville

William F. Galvin, BA, MSEd, CRT, RRT, CPFT
Assistant Professor, School of Allied
 Health
Program Director, Respiratory Care
 Program
Teaching Faculty, TIPS Program
Gwynedd-Mercy College
Gwynedd Valley, Pa.

Trish Goudie, RN, CNM, MSN
Dean and Associate Professor
College of Nursing
Montana State University – Northern
Havre

Grace G. Lewis, RN, MS, BC
Assistant Professor of Nursing
Georgia Baptist College of Nursing of
 Mercer University
Atlanta

Paul Keith Small, PhD
Professor of Biology
Chair of Science and Mathematics
 Division
Eureka (Ill.) College

Cheryl Westlake, RN, PhD, CS, PN
Assistant Professor
California State University Fullerton
Coordinator, Center of Excellence
Mission Hospital
Mission Viejo, Calif.

Robin R. Wilkerson, RN, PhD, BC
Associate Professor
University of Mississippi
Jackson

Kate Willcutts, MS, RD, CNSD
Surgery Nutrition Support/Instructor
School of Nursing
University of Virginia
Charlottesville

Foreword

Every health care professional requires a basic understanding of anatomy and physiology. However, the vast details associated with these subjects can be overwhelming at times, and you probably have moments when you need to double-check a critical fact about the structure and function of the human body. *Anatomy & Physiology Made Incredibly Easy*, Second Edition, summarizes this enormous amount of information into one resource that can be used to help you stay current while presenting the basic anatomic and physiologic principles in an easy-to-understand format. Through detailed diagrams and illustrations, you'll be able to visualize and conceptualize the information and perhaps even laugh a little along the way with a humor that's used to help emphasize important points.

The content of *Anatomy & Physiology Made Incredibly Easy* is logically organized, beginning with chapter 1, which provides an overview of cell structure, function, and cell division in the human body. This information, such as the DNA of a cell, serves as the building blocks for the more detailed examinations of the body systems that follow in later chapters. Chapters 2 and 3 build on this foundation by presenting the complexities of genetics and the body's chemical organization and processes—information that's fundamental to understanding the physiologic functions covered in the rest of the book.

Chapters 4 through 17 give a thorough overview of the integumentary, musculoskeletal, nervous, endocrine, cardiovascular, hematologic, immune, respiratory, gastrointestinal, urinary, and reproductive systems, including expanded coverage of complex topics, such as nutrition and metabolism; fluids, electrolytes, acids, and bases; and lactation.

Each chapter begins with the basics and breaks down complex concepts into easy-to-understand components. Key terms are italicized and defined throughout the text, making the book even easier to use. At the end of each chapter, a *Quick quiz* allows you to test your understanding of the information you just reviewed. And there's no need to flip back through the chapter to find out if you're right; the answers are provided with rationales to help with your learning.

This one-of a-kind book is loaded with anatomic illustrations, schematic representations, tables, and flow charts that complement and reinforce the written text. A special 16-page color section of anatomic illustrations provides even more in-depth coverage and helps you to better visualize anatomic structures, including the heart and the respiratory system.

New components and features make this book even easier to understand and more enjoyable to read. These new features include:
• *Incredibly Easy miniguide to physiology*—a new 16-page four-color section on normal physiologic processes, such as cardiac conduction and gas exchange, that complements the existing *Incredibly Easy miniguide to anatomy*
• *Senior moments*—explanations about how the normal aging process affects anatomy and physiology, a topic of growing importance given the rapid rise in the elderly population.

You'll also find these special graphics throughout the book that will alert you to important points:

 Zoom in — provides a closer look at anatomic structures you need to know

 Now I get it! — transforms complex elements of physiology into easy-to-digest explanations

 Body shop — breaks down the complex physiology of larger body structures and systems and shows how they all work together

 Memory jogger — reinforces learning through easy-to-remember anecdotes and mnemonics.

Whether you're in the classroom or in the field, *Anatomy & Physiology Made Incredibly Easy*, Second Edition, was designed with your needs in mind. Students will find text that's clearly presented, concise, and essential to learning the basics, designed to help them ace anatomy and physiology courses. Clinicians will find a handy reference that they will use again and again for quick reviews of numerous subjects encountered daily in clinical practice.

Joyce King, RN, FNP, CNM, PhD
Assistant Professor, Clinical
Emory University School of Nursing
Atlanta

Shrewsbury Health Library
Issue Receipt

Customer ID: S66***

Title: Assessment made incredibly easy /
Rushforth, Helen
ID: 30121005313489
Due: 30-APR-2018

Title: Anatomy and physiology made incredibly
easy / Bruck, Laura
ID: 30121005198005
Due: 30-APR-2018

Total items: 2
16-Apr-2018
Checked out: 3
Overdue: 0
Hold requests: 0
Ready for pickup: 0

Items that you already have on loan

Title: Critical care nursing made incredibly
easy! / Cutler, Lee
ID: T13272
Due: 14-May-2018

Thank you for using our services.

The human body

Just the facts

In this chapter, you'll learn:

♦ anatomic terms for direction, reference planes, body cavities, and body regions to help describe the locations of various body structures

♦ the structure of cells

♦ cell reproduction and energy generation

♦ four basic tissue types and their characteristics.

Anatomic terms

Anatomic terms describe directions within the body as well as the body's planes, cavities, and regions.

Directional terms

When navigating the body, directional terms help you determine the exact location of a structure.

Couples at odds

Generally, directional terms can be grouped in pairs of opposites:

• *Superior* and *inferior* mean above and below, respectively. For example, the shoulder is superior to the elbow, and the hand is inferior to the wrist.

• *Anterior* means toward the front of the body, and *posterior* means toward the back. *Ventral* is sometimes used instead of anterior, and *dorsal* is sometimes used instead of posterior.

> Locating body structures starts with directional terms, reference planes, cavities, and regions.

• *Medial* means toward the body's midline and *lateral* means away from it.
• *Proximal* and *distal* mean closest and farthest, respectively, to the point of origin (or to the trunk).
• *Superficial* and *deep* mean toward or at the body surface and farthest from it.

Memory jogger

To remember the meanings of **proximal** and **distal,** keep in mind that when something is in **proximity,** it's nearby. When something is **distant,** it's far away.

Reference planes

Reference planes are imaginary lines used to section the body and its organs. These lines run longitudinally, horizontally, and angularly.

The four major body reference planes are:

median sagittal

Body shop

Picturing body reference planes

Body reference planes are used to indicate the locations of body structures. Shown at right are the median sagittal, frontal, and transverse planes. An oblique plane—a slanted plane that lies between a horizontal plane and a vertical plane—isn't shown.

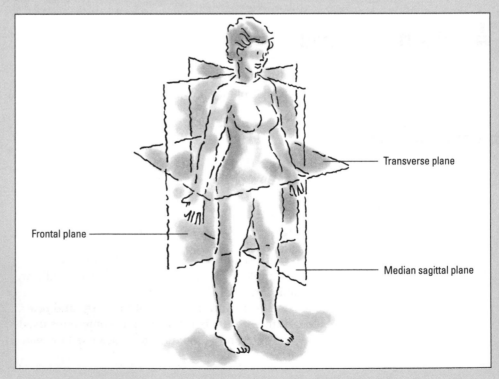

Transverse plane

Frontal plane

Median sagittal plane

frontal

 transverse

 oblique. (See *Picturing body reference planes.*)

Body cavities

Body cavities are spaces within the body that contain the internal organs. The *dorsal* and *ventral cavities* are the two major closed cavities — cavities without direct openings to the outside of the body. (See *Locating body cavities.*)

Dorsal cavity

The dorsal cavity is located in the posterior region of the body.

Body shop

Locating body cavities

The dorsal cavity, in the posterior region of the body, is divided into the cranial and vertebral cavities. The ventral cavity, in the anterior region, is divided into the thoracic and abdominopelvic cavities. These regions are shown in the illustration at right.

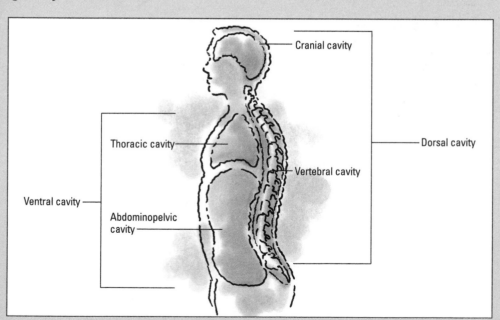

The think tank and backbone of the operation

The dorsal cavity is further subdivided into two cavities:
• The *cranial cavity* (also called the *calvaria*) encases the brain.
• The *vertebral cavity* (also called the *spinal cavity* or *vertebral canal*), formed by the vertebrae, encloses the spinal cord.

Ventral cavity

The ventral cavity occupies the anterior region of the trunk. This cavity is subdivided into the *thoracic cavity* and the *abdominopelvic cavity*.

Treasure chest

Surrounded by the ribs and chest muscles, the thoracic cavity refers to the space located superior to the abdominopelvic cavity. It's subdivided into the *pleural cavities* and the *mediastinum:*
• Each of the two *pleural cavities* contains a lung.
• The *mediastinum* houses the heart, large vessels of the heart, trachea, esophagus, thymus, lymph nodes, and other blood vessels and nerves.

We're located in the pleural cavities.

The bread basket and below

The abdominopelvic cavity has two regions, the *abdominal cavity* and the *pelvic cavity:*
• The *abdominal cavity* contains the stomach, intestines, spleen, liver, and other organs.
• The *pelvic cavity*, which lies inferior to the abdominal cavity, contains the bladder, some of the reproductive organs, and the rectum.

Other cavities

The body also contains an *oral cavity* (the mouth), a *nasal cavity* (located in the nose), *orbital cavities* (which house the eyes), *middle ear cavities* (which contain the small bones of the middle ear), and the *synovial cavities* (enclosed within the capsules surrounding freely moveable joints).

Body regions

Body regions are used to designate body areas that have special nerves or vascular supplies or those that perform special functions.

The guts of the matter

The most widely used body region terms are those that designate the sections of the abdomen. (See *Abdominal regions exposed.*) The abdomen has nine regions:

Body shop

Abdominal regions exposed

Here's an anterior view of the abdominal regions.

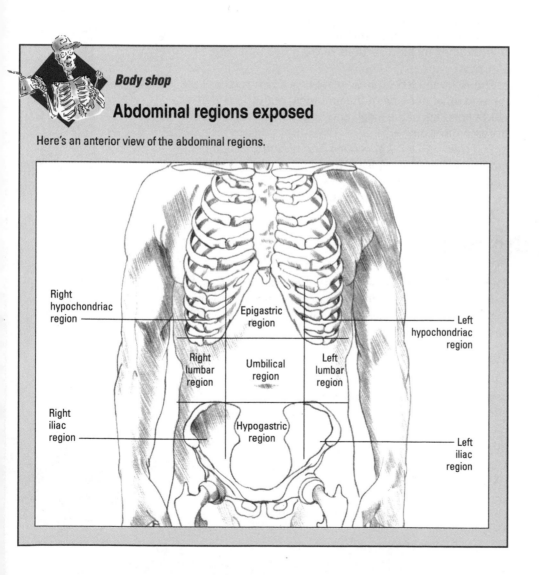

Right hypochondriac region

Epigastric region

Left hypochondriac region

Right lumbar region

Umbilical region

Left lumbar region

Right iliac region

Hypogastric region

Left iliac region

• The *umbilical region*, the area around the umbilicus, includes sections of the small and large intestines, inferior vena cava, and abdominal aorta.

• The *epigastric region*, superior to the umbilical region, contains most of the pancreas and portions of the stomach, liver, inferior vena cava, abdominal aorta, and duodenum.

• The *hypogastric region* (or pubic area), inferior to the umbilical region, houses a portion of the sigmoid colon, the urinary bladder and ureters, the uterus and ovaries (in females), and portions of the small intestine.

• The right and left *iliac regions* (or inguinal regions) are situated on either side of the hypogastric region. They include portions of the small and large intestines.

• The right and left *lumbar regions* (or loin regions) are located on either side of the umbilical region. They include portions of the small and large intestines and portions of the kidneys.

• The right and left *hypochondriac regions*, which reside on either side of the epigastric region, contain the diaphragm, portions of the kidneys, the right side of the liver, the spleen, and part of the pancreas.

Remember, each region has a specific nerve or vascular supply or performs a special function.

A look at the cell

The *cell* makes up the body's structure and serves as the basic unit of living matter. Human cells vary widely, ranging from the simple squamous epithelial cell to the highly specialized neuron.

The greatest regeneration

Generally, the simpler the cell, the greater its power to regenerate. The more specialized the cell, the weaker its regenerative power. Cells with greater regenerative power have shorter life spans than those with less regenerative power.

Sometimes simpler is better. The more simple I am, the more I can regenerate!

Cell structure

Cells are made up of three basic components:
• protoplasm

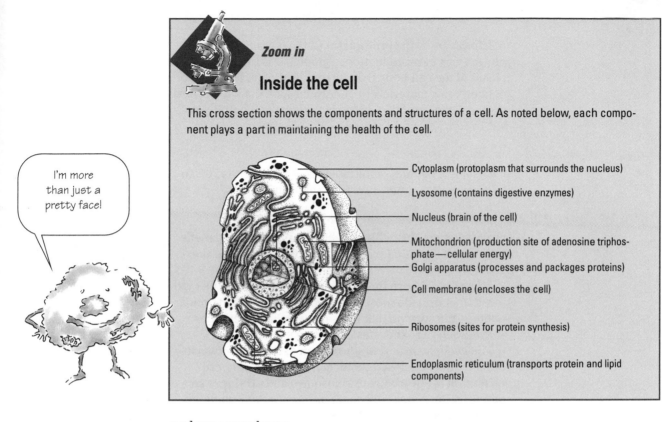

Zoom in

Inside the cell

This cross section shows the components and structures of a cell. As noted below, each component plays a part in maintaining the health of the cell.

Cytoplasm (protoplasm that surrounds the nucleus)

Lysosome (contains digestive enzymes)

Nucleus (brain of the cell)

Mitochondrion (production site of adenosine triphosphate—cellular energy)

Golgi apparatus (processes and packages proteins)

Cell membrane (encloses the cell)

Ribosomes (sites for protein synthesis)

Endoplasmic reticulum (transports protein and lipid components)

I'm more than just a pretty face!

- plasma membrane
- nucleus. (See *Inside the cell.*)

Protoplasm

Protoplasm, a viscous, translucent, watery material, is the primary component of plant and animal cells. It contains a large percentage of water, inorganic ions (such as potassium, calcium, magnesium, and sodium), and naturally occurring organic compounds (such as proteins, lipids, and carbohydrates).

Getting charged

The inorganic ions within protoplasm are called *electrolytes*. They regulate acid-base balance and control the amount of intracellular water. When these ions lose electrons (minute particles with a negative charge), they acquire a positive electrical charge. When they gain electrons, they acquire a negative electrical charge.

A pair of "plasms"

Nucleoplasm is the protoplasm of the cell's nucleus. It plays a part in reproduction. *Cytoplasm* is the protoplasm of the cell body that surrounds the nucleus. It converts raw materials to energy. It's also the site of most synthesizing activities. In the cytoplasm you'll find *cytosol*, *organelles*, and *inclusions*.

A cytosol sea

Cytosol is a viscous, semitransparent fluid that is 70% to 90% water. It contains proteins, salts, and sugars.

A lot to metabolize

Organelles are the cell's metabolic units. Each organelle performs a specific function to maintain the life of the cell:

Organelles are my metabolic units.

• *Mitochondria* are threadlike structures within the cytoplasm that provide most of the body's adenosine triphosphate—the enzyme that fuels many cellular activities.
• *Ribosomes* are the sites of protein synthesis.
• The *endoplasmic reticulum* is an extensive network of membrane-enclosed tubules. *Rough endoplasmic reticulum* is covered with ribosomes and produces certain proteins. *Smooth endoplasmic reticulum* contains enzymes that synthesize lipids.
• Each *Golgi apparatus* synthesizes carbohydrate molecules. These molecules combine with the proteins produced by rough endoplasmic reticulum to form secretory products such as lipoproteins.
• *Lysosomes* are digestive bodies that break down foreign or damaged material in cells. (See *Lysosomes at work.*)
• *Peroxisomes* contain *oxidases*, enzymes capable of reducing oxygen to hydrogen peroxide and hydrogen peroxide to water.
• *Cytoskeletal elements* form a network of protein structures.
• *Centrosomes* contain *centrioles*, short cylinders that are adjacent to the nucleus and take part in cell division.

Temps that don't do any work

Inclusions are nonfunctioning units in the cytoplasm that are commonly temporary. The pigment *melanin* in epithelial cells and the stored nutrient *glycogen* in liver cells are both examples of nonfunctioning units.

Now I get it!

Lysosomes at work

Lysosomes are the organelles responsible for digestion within a cell. Phagocytes assist in this process. Here's how lysosomes work.

Function of lysosomes
Lysosomes are digestive bodies that break down foreign or damaged material in cells. A membrane surrounds each lysosome and separates its digestive enzymes from the rest of the cytoplasm.

Breaking it down
The lysosomal enzymes digest matter brought into the cell by *phagocytes,* special cells that surround and engulf matter outside the cell and then transport it through the cell membrane. The membrane of the lysosome fuses with the membrane of the cytoplasmic spaces surrounding the phagocytized material; this fusion allows the lysosomal enzymes to digest the engulfed material.

Plasma membrane

The *plasma membrane* (cell membrane) is the gatekeeper of the cell. It serves as the cell's external boundary, separating it from other cells and from the external environment.

Checkpoint

Nothing gets by this semipermeable membrane without authorization from the nucleus. Roughly 75Å (3 ten-millionths of an inch) thick, it consists of a double layer of phospholipids with protein molecules.

Nucleus

The *nucleus* is the cell's mission control. It plays a role in cell growth, metabolism, and reproduction.

A nucleus may contain one or more *nucleoli* — a dark-staining structure that synthesizes *ribonucleic acid* (RNA). The nucleus also contains *chromosomes.* Chromosomes control cellular activity and direct protein synthesis through ribosomes in the cytoplasm. (For more information on chromosomes, see chapter 2, Genetics.)

DNA and RNA

Protein synthesis is essential for the growth of new tissue and the repair of damaged tissue. *Deoxyribonucleic acid* (DNA) carries genetic information and provides the blueprint for protein synthesis. RNA transfers this genetic information to the ribosomes, where protein synthesis occurs.

Touching all the bases

The basic structural unit of DNA is a *nucleotide*. Nucleotides consist of a phosphate group that is linked to a five-carbon sugar, *deoxyribose*, and joined to a nitrogen-containing compound called a *base*. Four different DNA bases exist:

 adenine (A)

 guanine (G)

 thymine (T)

cytosine (C).

We're complementary. That means we fit together perfectly.

Identifying rings

Adenine and *guanine* are double-ring compounds classified as *purines*. *Thymine* and *cytosine* are single-ring compounds classified as *pyrimidines*.

The chain gangs

DNA chains exist in pairs held together by weak chemical attractions between the nitrogen bases on adjacent chains. Because of the chemical shape of the bases, adenine bonds only with thymine and guanine bonds only with cytosine. Bases that can link with each other are called *complementary*.

Insider trading

RNA consists of nucleotide chains that differ slightly from the nucleotide chains found in DNA. Several types of RNA are involved in the transfer (to the ribosomes) of genetic information essential to protein synthesis. (See *Types of RNA*.)

Now I get it!

Types of RNA

There are three types of ribonucleic acid (RNA): ribosomal, messenger, and transfer. Each has its own specific function.

Ribosomal RNA

Ribosomal RNA is used to make ribosomes in the endoplasmic reticulum of the cytoplasm, where the cell produces proteins.

Messenger RNA

Messenger RNA directs the arrangement of amino acids to make proteins at the ribosomes. Its single strand of nucleotides is complementary to a segment of the deoxyribonucleic acid chain that contains instructions for protein synthesis. Its chains pass from the nucleus into the cytoplasm, attaching to ribosomes there.

Transfer RNA

Transfer RNA consists of short nucleotide chains, each of which is specific for an individual amino acid. Transfer RNA transfers the genetic code from messenger RNA for the production of a specific amino acid.

Cell reproduction

Cells are under a constant call to reproduce; it's either that or die. Cell division is how cells reproduce (or replicate) themselves; they achieve this through the process of *mitosis* or *meiosis*.

DNA does its thing

Before a cell divides, its chromosomes are duplicated. During this process, the double helix separates into two DNA chains. Each chain serves as a template for constructing a new chain. Individual DNA nucleotides are linked into new strands with bases complementary to those in the original.

Double double

In this way, two identical double helices are formed, each containing one of the original strands and a newly formed com-

I love creating a "new me."

Zoom in

DNA up close

Linked deoxyribonucleic acid (DNA) chains form a spiral structure, or *double helix*.

A spiral staircase

To understand linked DNA chains, imagine a spiral staircase. The deoxyribose and phosphate groups form the railings of the staircase, and the nitrogen base pairs (adenine and thymine, guanine and cytosine) form the steps.

Cell division

Each chain serves as a template for constructing a new chain. When a cell divides, individual DNA nucleotides are linked into new strands with bases complementary to those in the originals. In this way, two identical double helices are formed, each containing one of the original strands and a newly formed complementary strand. These double helices are duplicates of the original DNA chain.

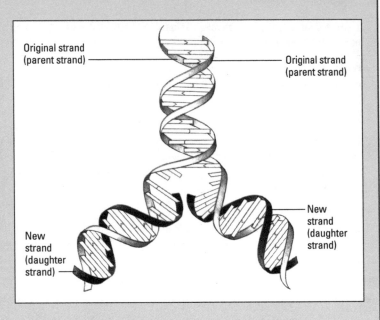

Original strand (parent strand)

Original strand (parent strand)

New strand (daughter strand)

New strand (daughter strand)

plementary strand. These double helices are duplicates of the original DNA chain. (See *DNA up close.*)

Mitosis

Mitosis is the equal division of material in the nucleus (*karyokinesis*) followed by division of the cell body (*cytokinesis*). It's the preferred mode of replication by all cells in the human body, except the gametes. Cell division occurs in five phases, an inactive phase called *interphase*, and four active phases:

 prophase

 metaphase

 anaphase

 telophase.

He may think he's better than me, but we have identical DNA!

Two daughters equal 46

Mitosis results in two daughter cells (exact duplicates), each containing 23 pairs of chromosomes — or 46 individual chromosomes. This number is the *diploid number*. (See *Divide and conquer: Five stages of mitosis*, page 14.)

Memory jogger

To help you remember the difference between haploid and diploid think of the prefix **di**- in **di**ploid. *Di*- means double, so diploid cells have double the number of chromosomes in a haploid cell.

Meiosis

Meiosis is reserved for gametes (ova and spermatozoa). This process intermixes genetic material between homologous chromosomes, producing four daughter cells, each with the *haploid number* of chromosomes (23, or half of the 46). Meiosis has two divisions separated by a resting phase.

First division

The first division has six phases and begins with one parent cell. When the first division ends, the result is two daughter cells — each containing the haploid (23) number of chromosomes.

Division 2, the sequel

The second division is a four-phase division that resembles mitosis. It starts with two new daughter cells, each containing the haploid number of chromosomes, and ends with four new haploid cells. In each cell, the two chromatids of each chromosome separate to form new daughter cells. However, because each cell entering the second division has only 23 chromosomes, each daughter cell formed has only 23 chromosomes. (See *Meiosis: Step-by-step*, page 15.)

Cellular energy generation

All cellular function depends on energy generation and transportation of substances within and among cells.

Cellular power

Adenosine triphosphate (ATP) serves as the chemical fuel for cellular processes. ATP consists of a nitrogen-containing compound (adenine) joined to a five-carbon

Now I get it!

Divide and conquer: Five stages of mitosis

Through the process of mitosis, the nuclear content of all body cells (except gametes) reproduces and divides. The result is the formation of two new daughter cells, each containing the diploid (46) number of chromosomes.

Interphase
During *interphase*, the nucleus and nuclear membrane are well defined, and the nucleolus is visible. As chromosomes replicate, each forms a double strand that remains attached at the center by a centromere.

Prophase
In *prophase*, the nucleolus disappears and the chromosomes become distinct. *Chromatids*, halves of each duplicated chromosome, remain attached by the centromere. Centrioles move to opposite sides of the cell and radiate spindle fibers.

Metaphase
Metaphase occurs when chromosomes line up randomly in the center of the cell between the spindles, along the *metaphase plate.* The centromere of each chromosome then replicates.

Anaphase
Anaphase is characterized by centromeres moving apart, pulling the separate chromatids (now called *chromosomes*) to opposite ends of the cell. The number of chromosomes at each end of the cell equals the original number.

Telophase
During *telophase,* the final stage of mitosis, a nuclear membrane forms around each nucleus and spindle fibers disappear. The cytoplasm compresses and divides the cell in half. Each new cell contains the diploid (46) number of chromosomes.

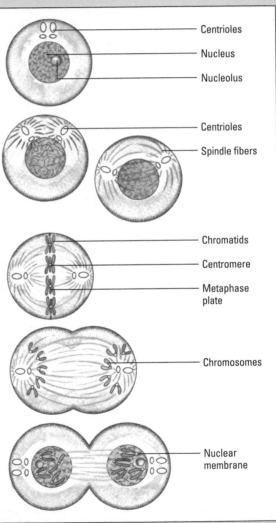

sugar (ribose), forming adenosine. Adenosine is joined to three phosphate (or triphosphate) groups. Chemical bonds between the first and second phosphate groups

Now I get it!

Meiosis: Step-by-step

Meiosis has two divisions that are separated by a resting phase. By the end of the first division, two daughter cells exist that each contain the haploid (23) number of chromosomes. When the second division ends, each of the two daughter cells from the first division divides, resulting in four daughter cells, each containing the haploid number of chromosomes.

First division
The first division has six phases. Here's what happens during each one.

Interphase
1. Chromosomes replicate, forming a double strand attached at the center by a centromere.
2. Chromosomes appear as an indistinguishable matrix within the nucleus.
3. Centrioles appear outside the nucleus.

Prophase I
1. The nucleolus and nuclear membrane disappear.
2. Chromosomes are distinct, with chromatids attached by the centromere.
3. Homologous chromosomes move close together and intertwine; exchange of genetic information (genetic recombination) may occur.
4. Centrioles separate and spindle fibers appear.

Metaphase I
1. Pairs of synaptic chromosomes line up randomly along the metaphase plate.
2. Spindle fibers attach to each chromosome pair.

Anaphase I
1. Synaptic pairs separate.
2. Spindle fibers pull homologous, double-stranded chromosomes to opposite ends of the cell.
3. Chromatids remain attached.

Telophase I
1. The nuclear membrane forms.
2. Spindle fibers and chromosomes disappear.
3. Cytoplasm compresses and divides the cell in half.
4. Each new cell contains the haploid (23) number of chromosomes.

Interkinesis
1. The nucleus and nuclear membrane are well defined.
2. The nucleolus is prominent, and each chromosome has two chromatids that don't replicate.

Second division
The second division closely resembles mitosis and is characterized by these four phases.

Prophase II
1. The nuclear membrane disappears.
2. Spindle fibers form.
3. Double-stranded chromosomes appear as thin threads.

Metaphase II
1. Chromosomes line up along the metaphase plate.
2. Centromeres replicate.

Anaphase II
1. Chromatids separate (now a single-stranded chromosome).
2. Chromosomes move away from each other to the opposite ends of the cell.

Telophase II
1. The nuclear membrane forms.
2. Chromosomes and spindle fibers disappear.
3. Cytoplasm compresses, dividing the cell in half.
4. Four daughter cells are created, each of which contains the haploid (23) number of chromosomes.

and between the second and third phosphate groups contain abundant energy.

The three R's

ATP needs to be converted to *adenosine diphosphate* (ADP) to produce energy. To understand this conversion, remember the three R's:
• *Rupture* — ATP is converted to ADP when the terminal high-energy phosphate bond ruptures.
• *Release* — Because the third phosphate is liberated, energy stored in the chemical bond is released.
• *Recycle* — Mitochondrial enzymes then reconvert ADP and the liberated phosphate to ATP. To obtain the energy needed for this reattachment, mitochondria oxidize food nutrients. This makes recycled ATP available again for energy production.

Movement within cells

Each cell interacts with body fluids through the interchange of substances.

Modes of transportation

Several transport methods — *diffusion, osmosis, active transport,* and *endocytosis* — move substances between cells and body fluids. In another method, *filtration,* fluids and dissolved substances are transferred across capillaries into *interstitial fluid* (fluid in the spaces between cells and tissues).

Diffusion

In *diffusion,* solutes move from an area of higher concentration to one of lower concentration. Eventually an equal distribution of solutes between the two areas occurs.

Go with the flow

Diffusion is a form of passive transport — no energy is required to make it happen; it just happens. It's kind of like fish traveling downstream. They just go with the flow.

No energy is required for diffusion. So I'll just go with the flow.

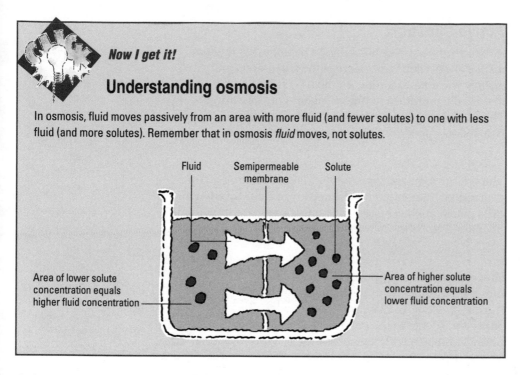

Now I get it!

Understanding osmosis

In osmosis, fluid moves passively from an area with more fluid (and fewer solutes) to one with less fluid (and more solutes). Remember that in osmosis *fluid* moves, not solutes.

Fluid · Semipermeable membrane · Solute

Area of lower solute concentration equals higher fluid concentration

Area of higher solute concentration equals lower fluid concentration

Advancing and declining rates

Several factors influence the rate of diffusion:
- *concentration gradient* — the greater the concentration gradient (the difference in particle concentration on either side of the plasma membrane), the faster the rate of diffusion
- *particle size* — the smaller the particles, the faster the rate of diffusion
- *lipid solubility* — the more lipid-soluble the particles are, the more rapidly they diffuse through the lipid layers of the cell membrane.

Osmosis

Osmosis is the passive movement of fluid across a membrane, from an area of lower solute concentration (comparatively *more* fluid) into an area of higher solute concentration (comparatively *less* fluid).

Enough is enough

Osmosis stops when enough fluid has moved through the membrane to equalize the solute concentration on both sides of the membrane. (See *Understanding osmosis*.)

Active transport

Active transport requires energy. Usually, this mechanism moves a substance across the cell membrane against the concentration gradient — from an area of lower concentration to one of higher concentration. Think of active transport as swimming upstream. When a fish swims upstream, it has to expend energy.

ATP at it again

The energy required for a solute to move against a concentration gradient comes from ATP. ATP is stored in all cells and supplies energy for solute movement in and out of cells.

It goes both ways

However, active transport also can move a substance with the concentration gradient. In this process, a carrier molecule in the cell membrane combines with the substance and transports it through the membrane, depositing it on the other side.

Active transport requires energy. As a cell, that means I need to fill up on ATP.

Endocytosis

Endocytosis is an active transport method in which, instead of passing through the cell membrane, a substance is engulfed by the cell. The cell surrounds the substance with part of the cell membrane. This part separates to form a *vacuole* (cavity) that moves to the cell's interior.

Gobbling up particles

Endocytosis involves either *phagocytosis* or *pinocytosis*. Phagocytosis refers to engulfment and ingestion of particles that are too large to pass through the cell membrane. Pinocytosis occurs only to engulf dissolved substances or small particles suspended in fluid.

Filtration

Fluid and dissolved substances also may move across a cell membrane by *filtration*.

Pressure is the point

In filtration, pressure (provided by capillary blood) is applied to a solution on one side of the cell membrane. The pressure forces fluid and dissolved particles through the membrane. The rate of filtration (how quickly substances pass through the membrane) depends on the amount of pressure. Filtration promotes the transfer of fluids and dissolved materials from the blood across the capillaries into the interstitial fluid.

A look at human tissue

Tissues are groups of cells that perform the same general function. The human body contains four basic types: *epithelial*, *connective*, *muscle*, and *nervous tissue*.

A crowd of us cells working together on the same function is called tissue.

Epithelial tissue

Epithelial tissue (epithelium) is a continuous cellular sheet that covers the body's surface, lines body cavities, and forms certain glands. Imagining a mummy wrapped in strips of cloth will give you some idea of how epithelial tissue covers the human body. (See *Distinguishing types of epithelial tissue*, page 20.)

Patrolling the borders

Some columnar epithelial cells in the lining of the intestines have vertical striations, forming a *striated border*. In the tubules of the kidneys, borders of columnar epithelial cells have tiny, brushlike structures (microvilli) called a *brush border*.

This hair isn't just for looks

Two common types of cells that form epithelial tissue are *stereociliated* and *ciliated epithelial cells*. The former line the epididymis and have long, piriform (pear-shaped) tufts. The latter possess *cilia*, fine hairlike protuberances. Cilia are larger than microvilli and move fluid and particles through the cavity of an organ.

Zoom in

Distinguishing types of epithelial tissue

Epithelial tissue (epithelium) is classified by the number of cell layers and the shape of surface cells. Some types of epithelium go through a process of desquamation (shedding of debris) and regenerate continuously by transformation of cells from deeper layers.

Identified by number of cell layers

Classified by number of cell layers, epithelium may be *simple* (one-layered), *stratified* (multilayered), or *pseudostratified* (one-layered but appearing to be multilayered).

Classified by shape

If classified by shape, epithelium may be *squamous* (containing flat surface cells), *columnar* (containing tall, cylindrical surface cells), or *cuboidal* (containing cube-shaped surface cells).

The top left illustration below shows how the basement membrane of simple squamous epithelium joins the epithelium to underlying connective tissues. The remaining illustrations show the five other types of epithelial tissue.

Simple squamous epithelium
Single layer of flattened cells with disc-shaped nuclei

Simple columnar epithelium
Single layer of tall cells with oval nuclei

Stratified squamous epithelium
Basal cells that are cuboidal or columnar

Simple cuboidal epithelium
Single layer of cubelike cells

Stratified columnar epithelium
Superficial cells that are elongated and columnar

Pseudostratified columnar epithelium
Cells of different height with nuclei at different levels

Endothelium

Epithelial tissue with a single layer of squamous cells attached to a basement membrane is called *endothelium*.

Such tissue lines the heart, lymphatic vessels, and blood vessels.

Glandular epithelium

Organs that produce secretions consist of a special type of epithelium called *glandular epithelium*.

The secret is in how it secretes

Glands are classified as exocrine or endocrine according to how they secrete their products:
• *Endocrine glands* release their secretions into the blood or lymph. For instance, the medulla of the adrenal gland secretes epinephrine and norepinephrine into the bloodstream.
• *Exocrine glands* discharge their secretions into ducts that lead to external or internal surfaces. One example is the sweat glands, which secrete sweat onto the surface of the skin.

Mixing it up

Mixed glands contain both endocrine and exocrine cells. The pancreas is a mixed gland. It contains alpha and beta cells (in the islets of Langerhans). These endocrine cells produce glucagon and insulin, respectively.

Connective tissue

Connective tissue — a category that includes bone, cartilage, and adipose (fatty) tissue — binds together and supports body structures. Connective tissue is classified as *loose* or *dense*.

Cut loose

Loose (areolar) connective tissue has large spaces that separate the fibers and cells. It contains a lot of intercellular fluid.

Dense tissue issues

Dense connective tissue provides structural support and has greater fiber concentration. Dense tissue is further subdivided into dense regular and dense irregular connective tissue:
• *Dense regular* connective tissue consists of tightly packed fibers arranged in a consistent pattern. It includes

tendons, ligaments, and *aponeuroses* (flat fibrous sheets that attach muscles to bones or other tissues).
• *Dense irregular* connective tissue has tightly packed fibers arranged in an inconsistent pattern. It's found in the dermis, submucosa of the GI tract, fibrous capsules, and fasciae.

Suppose it's adipose

Commonly called *fat, adipose tissue* is a specialized type of loose connective tissue where a single lipid (fat) droplet occupies most of each cell. Widely distributed subcutaneously, it acts as insulation to conserve body heat, as a cushion for internal organs, and as a storage depot for excess food and reserve supplies of energy.

What happened to your adipose tissue?

Tissue?! I don't even know you!

Muscle tissue

Muscle tissue consists of muscle cells with a generous blood supply. Muscle cells measure up to several centimeters long and have an elongated shape that enhances their *contractility* (ability to contract).

The tissues at issue

There are three basic types of muscle tissue:
• *Striated muscle tissue* gets its name from its striped, or striated, appearance; it contracts voluntarily.
• *Cardiac muscle tissue* is sometimes classified as striated because it too is composed of striated tissue. However, it differs from other striated muscle tissue in two ways: its fibers are separate cellular units that don't contain many nuclei, and it contracts involuntarily.
• *Smooth-muscle tissue* consists of long, spindle-shaped cells and lacks the striped pattern of striated tissue. Its activity is stimulated by the autonomic nervous system and isn't under voluntary control.

Wall tissue paper

Smooth-muscle tissue lines the walls of many internal organs and other structures, including the respiratory passages from the trachea to the alveolar ducts, the urinary and genital ducts, the arteries and veins, the larger lymphatic trunks, the intestines, the arrectores pilorum, and the iris and ciliary body of the eye.

Irritable!?
I'll show you irritable!

Nervous tissue

The main function of *nervous tissue* is communication. Its primary properties are *irritability* (the capacity to react to various physical and chemical agents) and *conductivity* (the ability to transmit the resulting reaction from one point to another).

Nervous tissue specialists

Neurons are highly specialized cells that generate and conduct nerve impulses. A typical neuron consists of a cell body with cytoplasmic extensions — numerous *dendrites* on one pole and a single *axon* on the opposite pole. These extensions allow the neuron to conduct impulses over long distances.

Protecting neurons

Neuroglia form the support structure of nervous tissue, insulating and protecting neurons. They're found only in the central nervous system.

Quick quiz

1.   The reference plane that divides the body lengthwise into right and left regions is the:
    A.   frontal plane.
    B.   sagittal plane.
    C.   transverse plane.
    D.   oblique plane.

Answer: B. Imaginary lines called reference planes are used to section the body. The sagittal plane runs lengthwise and divides the body into right and left regions.

2.   The structure that plays the biggest role in cellular function is the:
    A.   nucleus.
    B.   Golgi apparatus.
    C.   ribosome.
    D.   mitochondrion.

Answer: A. Serving as the cell's control center, the nucleus plays a role in cell growth, metabolism, and reproduction.

3. The four basic types of tissue that the human body contains are:
- A. muscle, cartilage, glandular, and connective tissue.
- B. bone, cartilage, glands, and adipose tissue.
- C. loose, dense connective, dense regular, and dense irregular tissue.
- D. epithelial, connective, muscle, and nervous tissue.

Answer: D. Tissues are groups of cells with the same general function. The human body contains four basic types of tissue: epithelial, connective, muscle, and nervous tissue.

4. Meiosis ends when:
- A. two new daughter cells form, each with the haploid number of chromosomes.
- B. one daughter cell forms and is an exact copy of the original.
- C. four new daughter cells form, each with the haploid number of chromosomes.
- D. four new daughter cells form, each with the diploid number of chromosomes.

Answer: C. Meiosis comes to completion with the end of telophase II. The result is four daughter cells, each of which contains the haploid (23) number of chromosomes.

Scoring

☆☆☆   If you answered all four questions correctly, fantastic! You're well on your way to a fantastic voyage through the human body.

☆☆   If you answered three questions correctly, all right! You're in for some smooth sailing. Pretty soon you'll know the body inside and out.

☆   If you answered fewer than three questions correctly, buck up, camper. With fifteen more quick quizzes, you'll conquer this body of knowledge in no time.

2

Genetics

Just the facts

In this chapter, you'll learn:

♦ the way traits are transmitted

♦ the role of chromosomes and genes in heredity

♦ factors that determine trait predominance

♦ causes of genetic defects.

A look at genetics

Genetics is the study of heredity—the passing of traits from biological parents to their children. People inherit not only physical traits, such as eye color, but also biochemical and physiologic traits, including the tendency to develop certain diseases. Genetic information is carried in *genes*, which are strung together on the *deoxyribonucleic acid* (DNA) double helix to form chromosomes.

Family inheritance

Parents transmit inherited traits to their offspring in germ cells, or *gametes*. There are two types of human gametes: eggs (ova) and sperm (spermatozoa). The traits a person inherits are determined at fertilization, when an ovum and a sperm unite.

Chromosomes

The nucleus of each germ cell contains structures called *chromosomes*. Each chromosome contains a strand of genetic material called *DNA*. DNA is a long molecule that's made up of thousands of segments called *genes*. These

Your genes determine how you look, how your body functions, and even whether you're prone to disease.

genes carry each trait that a person inherits, ranging from blood type to toe shape. Chromosomes exist in pairs except in the germ cells.

Counting chromosomes

A human ovum contains 23 chromosomes. A sperm also contains 23 chromosomes, each similar in size and shape to a chromosome in the ovum. When an ovum and a sperm unite, the corresponding chromosomes pair up. The result is a fertilized cell with 46 chromosomes (23 pairs) in its nucleus.

Gen XX (or XY)

Of the 23 pairs of chromosomes in each living human cell, the two sex chromosomes of the 23rd pair determine a person's gender. The other 22 pairs, called *autosomes*, have no effect on gender.

In a female, both sex chromosomes are relatively large and each is designated by the letter X. In a male, one sex chromosome is an X chromosome and one is a smaller chromosome, designated by the letter Y.

Each gamete produced by a male contains either an X or a Y chromosome. Each gamete produced by a female contains only an X chromosome. When a sperm with an X chromosome fertilizes an ovum, the offspring is female (two X chromosomes). When a sperm with a Y chromosome fertilizes an ovum, the offspring is male (one X and one Y chromosome).

Dividing the family assets

Ova and sperm are formed by a cell-division process called *meiosis*. In meiosis, each of the 23 pairs of chromosomes in a cell splits. The cell then divides, and each new cell (an ovum or sperm) receives one set of 23 chromosomes. (See chapter 1, The human body, page 13, for more information on meiosis.)

Genes

Genes are segments of a DNA chain, arranged in sequence on a chromosome. This sequence determines the properties of a cell.

The genome at a glance

The human genome is made up of a set of very long deoxyribonucleic acid (DNA) molecules, one for each chromosome. DNA has four different chemical building blocks, called *bases*. Each human genome contains about 3 billion of these bases, arranged in an order that's unique for each person. Increasing its complexity, arrayed along the DNA molecules are over 30,000 genes.

Consider its size: If the DNA sequence of the human genome were compiled in books, the equivalent of 200 volumes the size of the Manhattan telephone book (at 1,000 pages each) would be needed to hold it all.

If I were to read out loud the 3 billion bases in just one genome, it would take 9½ years.

Locus pocus

The location of a specific gene on a chromosome is called the *gene locus*. The locus of each gene is specific and doesn't vary from person to person. This allows each of the thousands of genes in an ovum to join the corresponding genes from a sperm when the chromosomes pair up at fertilization.

How do I look?

The genetic information stored at a locus of a gene determines the genetic constitution—or *genotype*—of a person. The detectable, outward manifestation of a genotype is called the *phenotype*.

I may look delicate, but I have a strong genotype.

The human genome

A complete set of chromosomes, containing all the genetic information for one person, is called a *genome*. (See *The genome at a glance*.)

The 411 on genes

For several years, scientists intensely studied the human genome to determine the entire sequence of each DNA molecule and the location and identity of all genes. The project was successfully completed in April 2003.

Catching the culprit

Genetic sequencing information allows doctors to identify the causes of disease rather than simply treating symptoms. Other benefits include future development of more specific diagnostic tests, the formation of new therapies, and methods for avoiding conditions that trigger disease.

In addition, doctors can now test patients for a gene error, present in 1 out of 500 people, that indicates a 60% chance of developing colon cancer. Similarly, women with family histories of breast or ovarian cancer can be tested for genetic predispositions to those diseases. Researchers are also seeking genes associated with dozens of other diseases, including chronic conditions such as asthma and diabetes.

It only takes one bad gene to spoil a gene pool party.

Trait predominance

Each parent contributes one set of chromosomes (and therefore one set of genes) to their offspring. Therefore, every offspring has two genes for every locus (location on the chromosome) on the autosomal chromosomes.

Variation is the spice of life

Some characteristics, or traits, are determined by one gene that may have many variants. Variations of the same gene are called *alleles*. A person who has identical alleles on each chromosome is *homozygous* for that trait; if the alleles are different, they're said to be *heterozygous*. Other traits — called *polygenic traits* — require the interaction of more than one gene.

Autosomal inheritance

On autosomal chromosomes, one allele may exert more influence in determining a specific trait. This is called the *dominant gene*. The less influential allele is called the *recessive gene*. Offspring express the trait of a dominant allele if both, or only one, chromosome in a pair carries it. For a recessive allele to be expressed, both chromosomes must carry identical alleles. (See *How genes express themselves*.)

Sex-linked inheritance

The X and Y chromosomes are the sex chromosomes. The X chromosome is much larger than the Y. Therefore, males (who have XY chromosomes) have less genetic material than females (who have XX chromosomes), which means they have only one copy of most genes on

Now I get it!

How genes express themselves

Genes account for inherited traits. *Gene expression* refers to a gene's effect on cell structure or function; however, the effects vary with the gene.

Dominant genes

If genes could speak, dominant genes would be loud and garrulous, dominating every conversation! Dominant genes (such as the one for dark hair) can be expressed and transmitted to the offspring even if only one parent possesses the gene.

Recessive genes

Unlike dominant genes, recessive genes prefer to hide their light under a bushel basket. A recessive gene (such as the one for blond hair) is expressed only when both parents transmit it to the offspring.

Codominant genes

Firm believers in equality, codominant genes (such as the genes that direct specific types of hemoglobin synthesis in red blood cells) allow expression of both alleles.

Sex-linked genes

Sex-linked genes are carried on sex chromosomes. Almost all appear on the X chromosome and are recessive. In the male, sex-linked genes behave like dominant genes because no second X chromosome exists.

the X chromosome. Inheritance of those genes is called *X-linked*, or *sex-linked*, *inheritance*.

Unequal X-change

A woman transmits one copy of each X-linked gene to each of her children, male or female. Because a man transmits an X chromosome only to his female children (male children receive a Y chromosome), he transmits X-linked genes only to his daughters, never his sons.

Multifactorial inheritance

Multifactorial inheritance reflects the interaction of at least two abnormal genes or the influence of environmental factors.

Raising the bar

Height is a classic example of a multifactorial trait. In general, the height of an offspring peaks between the heights of the two parents. However, nutritional patterns, health care, and other environmental factors also influence development of such traits as height. A better-nourished, healthier child of two short parents may be taller than either parent.

When it all comes together

Some diseases also have genetic predispositions for multifactorial inheritance; that is, the gene for a disease might be expressed only under certain environmental conditions.

Factors that may contribute to multifactorial inheritance include:
- maternal age
- use of drugs, alcohol, or hormones by either parent
- maternal smoking
- maternal or paternal exposure to radiation
- maternal infection during pregnancy
- preexisting diseases in the mother
- nutritional factors
- general maternal or paternal health
- maternal-fetal blood incompatibility
- inadequate prenatal care.

Good nutrition, proper health care, and other environmental factors can influence how a gene expresses itself.

Genetic defects

Genetic defects are defects that result from changes to genes or chromosomes. They're categorized as either autosomal disorders, sex-linked disorders, or multifactorial disorders. Some defects arise spontaneously, whereas others may be caused by environmental teratogens. *Teratogens* are environmental agents (such as infectious toxins, maternal diseases, drugs, chemicals, and physical agents) that can cause structural or functional defects in a developing fetus. They may also cause spontaneous abortion, complications during labor and delivery, hidden defects in later development (such as cognitive or behavioral problems), and benign or cancerous tumors.

Permanent change in plans

A permanent change in genetic material is known as a *mutation*. Mutations can result from exposure to radiation, certain chemicals, or viruses. They may also happen spontaneously and can occur anywhere in the genome.

Every cell has built-in defenses against genetic damage. However, if a mutation isn't identified or repaired, it may produce a new trait that can be transmitted to offspring. Some mutations produce no effect, others change the expression of a trait, and others can even change the way a cell functions. Some mutations cause serious or deadly defects, such as congenital anomalies and cancer.

Autosomal disorders

In autosomal disorders, an error occurs at a single gene site on the DNA strand. Single-gene disorders are inherited in clearly identifiable patterns that are the same as those seen in inheritance of normal traits. Because every person has 22 pairs of autosomes and only 1 pair of sex chromosomes, most hereditary disorders are caused by autosomal defects.

The assertive type

Autosomal dominant transmission involves transmission of an abnormal gene that's dominant. Autosomal dominant disorders usually affect male and female offspring equally. Children with one affected parent have a 50% chance of being affected.

Passive-aggressive behavior

Autosomal recessive inheritance involves transmission of a recessive gene that's abnormal. Autosomal recessive disorders also usually affects male and female offspring equally. If both parents are affected, all their offspring will be affected. If both parents are unaffected but carry the defective gene, each child has a 25% chance of being affected. If only one parent is affected, none of the offspring will be affected, but all will carry the defective gene. If one parent is affected and the other is a carrier, 50% of their children will be affected. Because of this transmission pattern, autosomal recessive disorders may occur even when there's no family history of the disease.

Sex-linked disorders

Genetic disorders caused by genes located on the sex chromosomes are termed *sex-linked disorders*.

X calls the shots

Most sex-linked disorders are controlled by genes on the X chromosome, usually as recessive traits. Because males have only one X chromosome, a single X-linked recessive gene can cause disease to be exhibited in a male. Females receive two X chromosomes, so they may be homozygous for a disease allele (and exhibit the disease), homozygous for a normal allele (and neither have nor carry the disease), or heterozygous (carry, but not exhibit, the disease).

Most people who express X-linked recessive traits are males with unaffected parents. In rare cases, the father is affected and the mother is a carrier. All daughters of an affected male are carriers. An affected male never transmits the trait to his son. Unaffected male children of a female carrier don't transmit the disorder.

Most people who have X-linked recessive disorders are males. That's because males have only one X chromosome. Females have a second X chromosome that overpowers the "diseased" X.

Evidence in history

With X-linked dominant inheritance, evidence of the inherited trait usually exists in the family history. A person with the abnormal trait must have one affected parent. If the father has an X-linked dominant disorder, all of his daughters and none of his sons will be affected. If a mother has an X-linked dominant disorder, each of her children has a 50% chance of being affected.

Multifactorial disorders

Most multifactorial disorders result from a number of genes and environmental influences acting together. In polygenic inheritance, each gene has a small additive effect and the combination of genetic errors is unpredictable. Multifactorial disorders can result from a less-than-optimum expression of many different genes, not from a specific error.

Mixing it up

Some multifactorial disorders are apparent at birth, such as cleft lip, cleft palate, congenital heart disease, anencephaly, clubfoot, and myelomeningocele. Others, such as type II diabetes mellitus, hypertension, hyperlipidemia, most autoimmune diseases, and many cancers, don't appear until later. Environmental factors most likely influence the development of multifactorial disorders during adulthood.

Chromosome defects

Aberrations in chromosome structure or number cause a class of disorders called *congenital anomalies*, or *birth defects*. Genetic aberrations include the loss, addition, or rearrangement of genetic material.

Most clinically significant chromosome aberrations arise during meiosis, an incredibly complex process that can go wrong in many ways. Potential contributing factors include maternal age, radiation, and use of some therapeutic or recreational drugs.

Unequally yoked

Translocation, the relocation of a segment of a chromosome to a nonhomologous chromosome, occurs when chromosomes split apart and rejoin in an abnormal arrangement. The cells still have a normal amount of genetic material, so often there are no visible abnormalities. However, the children of parents with translocated chromosomes may have serious genetic defects, such as monosomies or trisomies.

A *monosomy* is a condition in which the number of chromosomes present is one less than normal; an autosomal monosomy is incompatible with life. The presence of an extra chromosome is called a *trisomy*. A mixture of both trisomic and normal cells results in *mosaicism* (two or more cell lines in the same person). The effects of mosaicism depend on the number and location of abnormal cells.

Breaking up is hard to do

During both meiosis and mitosis, chromosomes normally separate in a process called *disjunction*. Failure to separate, called *nondisjunction*, causes an unequal distribution of chromosomes between the two resulting cells. If nondisjunction occurs soon after fertilization, it may affect all the resulting cells. The incidence of nondisjunction increases with parental age. (See *Chromosomal disjunction and nondisjunction*, page 34.)

Now I get it!

Chromosomal disjunction and nondisjunction

These illustrations show disjunction and nondisjunction of an ovum. When disjunction proceeds normally, fertilization with a normal sperm results in a zygote with the correct number of chromosomes. In nondisjunction, the duplicating chromosomes fail to separate; the result is one trisomic cell and one monosomic cell.

Quick quiz

1. What's the total number of chromosomes in a fertilized cell?

    A.   12
    B.   23
    C.   46
    D.   52

Answer: C. There are 46 chromosomes (23 pairs) in the nucleus of a fertilized cell.

2. According to genetic theory, if a child has blond hair, this must mean:

    A.   both parents transmit the gene for blond hair.
    B.   one parent transmits the gene for blond hair.
    C.   one grandparent has blond hair.
    D.   neither parent has the gene for blond hair.

Answer: A. Because the trait for blond hair is a recessive gene, it's only expressed when both parents transmit it to the offspring.

3. The presence of an extra chromosome is called:

    A.   monosomy.
    B.   trisomy.
    C.   mosaicism.
    D.   nondisjunction.

Answer: B. Trisomy is the presence of an extra chromosome; it results from nondisjunction.

4. Which of the following definitions applies to the term *mutation?*

    A.   An environmental agent responsible for a genetic defect
    B.   A permanent change in genetic material
    C.   Interaction of at least two abnormal genes
    D.   Expression of a recessive gene in an offspring

Answer: B. A mutation is a permanent change in genetic material that may result from exposure to radiation, certain chemicals, or viruses. Mutations may also occur spontaneously.

5. A child has brown eyes and brown hair. This description reveals the child's:

A. phenotype.
B. genotype.
C. genome.
D. autosomes.

Answer: A. Phenotype refers to the outward, detectable manifestation of a person's genetic makeup or genotype.

Scoring

☆☆☆ If you answered all five questions correctly, excellent! When it comes to genetics, you're a gene-ius.

☆☆ If you answered four questions correctly, good job! Your understanding of genetics is definitely dominant.

☆ If you answered fewer than four questions correctly, don't worry. Another look at the chapter may help to X-plain Y.

Chemical organization

Just the facts

In this chapter, you'll learn:

♦ the chemical composition of the body

♦ the structure of an atom

♦ differences between inorganic and organic compounds.

A look at body chemistry

The human body is composed of chemicals; in fact, all of its activities are chemical in nature. To understand the human body and its functions, you must understand chemistry.

Comes down to chemistry

The chemical level is the simplest and most important level of structural organization. Without the proper chemicals in the proper amounts, body cells — and eventually the body itself — would die.

Without chemicals in the proper amounts, I would die.

Principles of chemistry

Every cell contains thousands of different chemicals that constantly interact with one another. Differences in chemical composition differentiate types of body tissue. Furthermore, the blueprints of heredity (deoxyribonucleic acid [DNA] and ribonucleic acid [RNA]) are encoded in chemical form.

What's the matter?

Matter is anything that has mass and occupies space. It may be a solid, liquid, or gas.

Energetic types

Energy is the capacity to do work—to put mass into motion. It may be *potential energy* (stored energy) or *kinetic energy* (the energy of motion). Types of energy include chemical, electrical, and radiant.

Chemical composition

An *element* is matter that can't be broken down into simpler substances by normal chemical reactions. All forms of matter are composed of chemical elements. Each of the chemical elements in the periodic table has a chemical symbol. For example, N is the chemical symbol for nitrogen. (See *Understanding elements and compounds.*)

It's elementary

Carbon, hydrogen, nitrogen, and oxygen account for 96% of the body's total weight. Calcium and phosphorus account for another 2.5%. (See *What's a body made of?* page 40.)

Atomic structure

An *atom* is the smallest unit of matter that can take part in a chemical reaction. Atoms of a single type constitute an element.

Subatomic particles

Each atom has a dense central core called a *nucleus*, plus one or more surrounding energy layers called *electron shells.* Atoms consist of three basic subatomic particles: *protons, neutrons,* and *electrons.*

Weighing in

A proton weighs nearly the same as a neutron, and a proton and a neutron each weigh 1,836 times as much as an electron.

Now I get it!

Understanding elements and compounds

It can be confusing to understand the difference between elements and compounds. The best way to remember the difference is to understand how atoms combine to form each.

Get at them atoms
A single atom constitutes an element. Thus, an atom of hydrogen is the element hydrogen. Now, here's the confusing part: An element can also be composed of more than one atom—a molecule.

Molecules: Two (or more) of the same
A molecule is a combination of two or more atoms. If these atoms are the same—that is, all the same element (such as all hydrogen atoms)—they're considered a *molecule* of that element (a molecule of hydrogen).

Compounds: Where the different come together
If the atoms combined are different—that is, different elements (such as a carbon atom and an oxygen atom)—the molecule formed is a *compound* (such as the compound CO, or carbon monoxide).

Yep. I'm an atom — the smallest unit of matter that can take part in a chemical reaction.

We're atoms that are joined together to make a molecule. We're the same, so we're a molecule of an element.

I know we just met, but I think we'll make a beautiful compound together.

Protons

Protons (p+) are closely packed particles in the atom's nucleus that have a positive charge. Each element has a distinct number of protons.

Positive thinking

An element's number of protons determines its *atomic number* and positive charge. For example, all carbon atoms—and *only* carbon atoms—have 6 protons; therefore, the atomic number of carbon is 6 (6p+).

Body shop

What's a body made of?

This chart shows the chemical elements of the human body in descending order from most to least plentiful.

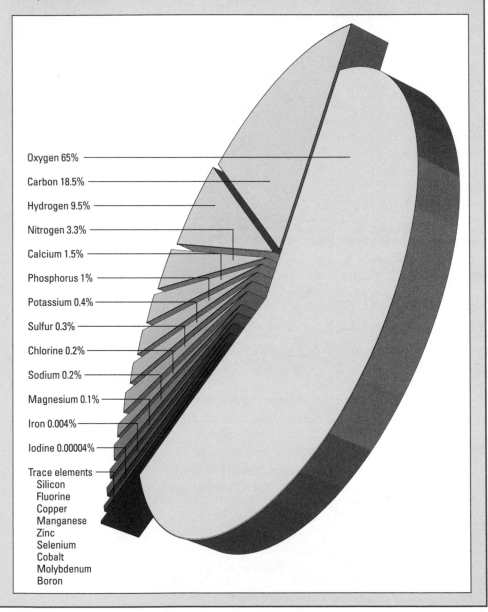

Oxygen 65%
Carbon 18.5%
Hydrogen 9.5%
Nitrogen 3.3%
Calcium 1.5%
Phosphorus 1%
Potassium 0.4%
Sulfur 0.3%
Chlorine 0.2%
Sodium 0.2%
Magnesium 0.1%
Iron 0.004%
Iodine 0.00004%
Trace elements
  Silicon
  Fluorine
  Copper
  Manganese
  Zinc
  Selenium
  Cobalt
  Molybdenum
  Boron

With all that oxygen, it's a wonder I don't just float away.

Neutrons

Neutrons (n) are uncharged, or neutral, particles in the atom's nucleus.

Mass numbers

An atom's *atomic mass number* is distinct from its atomic number. The atomic mass number is the sum of the number of protons and neutrons in the nucleus of an atom. You can also think of the atomic mass number as the sum of the masses of protons and neutrons. For example, helium, with two protons and two neutrons, has an atomic mass number of four.

Isolating the isotopes

Not all the atoms of an element necessarily have the same number of neutrons. An *isotope* is a form of an atom that has a different number of neutrons and, therefore, a different atomic weight.

A weighty matter

Understanding isotopes is a key to another important concept, *atomic weight*. An atom's atomic weight is the average of the relative weights (atomic mass numbers) of all the element's isotopes. (Recall that isotopes are different atomic forms of the same element that vary in the number of neutrons they contain.)

Electrons

Electrons (e-) are negatively charged particles that orbit the nucleus in electron shells. They play a key role in chemical bonds and reactions.

Staying neutral

The number of electrons in an atom equals the number of protons in its nucleus. The electrons' negative charges cancel out the protons' positive charges, making atoms electrically neutral.

Shell games

Electrons circle the nucleus in *shells* or concentric circles. Each electron shell can hold a maximum number of electrons and represents a specific energy level. The innermost shell can accommodate two electrons at most, whereas the outermost shells can hold many more.

An atom with single (unpaired) electrons orbiting in its outermost electron shell can be chemically *active* — that is, able to take part in chemical reactions. An atom with an outer shell that contains only pairs of electrons is chemically inactive, or *stable*.

The value of valence

An atom's *valence* (its ability to combine with other atoms) equals the number of unpaired electrons in its outer shell. For example, sodium (Na+) has a plus-one valence because its outer shell contains an unpaired electron.

It takes energy to bind atoms together. Breaking the bond releases energy.

Chemical bonds

A *chemical bond* is a force of attraction that binds a molecule's atoms together. Formation of a chemical bond usually requires energy. Breakup of a chemical bond usually releases energy.

The name's bond...

Several types of chemical bonds exist:
• A *hydrogen bond* occurs when two atoms associate with a hydrogen atom. Oxygen and nitrogen, for instance, commonly form hydrogen bonds.
• An *ionic* (electrovalent) *bond* occurs when valence electrons transfer from one atom to another.
• A *covalent bond* forms when atoms share pairs of valence electrons. (See *Picturing ionic and covalent bonds.*)

Chemical reactions

A *chemical reaction* involves unpaired electrons in the outer shells of atoms. In this reaction, one of two events occurs:

☞ Unpaired electrons from the outer shell of one atom transfer to the outer shell of another atom.

✌ One atom shares its unpaired electrons with another atom.

How will they react?

Energy, particle concentration, speed, and orientation determine whether a chemical reaction will occur. The four basic types of chemical reactions are *synthesis*, *decom-*

Now I get it!

Picturing ionic and covalent bonds

A chemical bond is a force of attraction that binds the atoms of a molecule together. Let's examine ionic and covalent bonds.

Ionic bonds

In an ionic bond, an electron is transferred from one atom to another. By forces of attraction, an electron is transferred from a sodium (Na) atom to a chlorine (Cl) atom. The result is a molecule of sodium chloride (NaCl).

Sodium atom (Na)   11+   Chlorine atom (Cl)   17+

Sodium ion (Na+)   11+   Chlorine ion (Cl−)   17+

Covalent bonds

In a covalent bond, atoms share a pair of electrons. This is what happens when two hydrogen (H) atoms form a covalent bond.

Hydrogen atom   +   Hydrogen atom   →   Hydrogen molecule (H_2)

position, exchange, and *reversible reactions.* (See *Comparing chemical reactions,* page 44.)

Inorganic and organic compounds

Although most biomolecules (molecules produced by living cells) form *organic compounds,* or compounds containing carbon, some form *inorganic compounds,* or compounds without carbon.

Now I get it!

Comparing chemical reactions

When chemical reactions occur, they involve unpaired electrons in the outer shells of atoms. Here are the four basic types of chemical reactions.

Synthesis reaction (anabolism)
A synthesis reaction combines two or more substances (reactants) to form a new, more complex substance (product). This results in a chemical bond.

$$A + B \rightarrow AB$$

Decomposition reaction (catabolism)
In a decomposition reaction, a substance decomposes, or breaks down, into two or more simpler substances, leading to the breakdown of a chemical bond.

$$AB \rightarrow A + B$$

Exchange reaction
An exchange reaction is a combination of a decomposition and a synthesis reaction. This reaction occurs when two complex substances decompose into simpler substances. The simple substances then join (through synthesis) with different simple substances to form new complex substances.

$$AB + CD \rightarrow A + B + C + D \rightarrow AD + BC$$

Reversible reaction
In a reversible reaction, the product reverts to its original reactants, and vice versa. Reversible reactions may require special conditions, such as heat or light.

$$A + B \leftrightarrow AB$$

Inorganic compounds

Inorganic compounds are usually small and include water and *electrolytes* — inorganic acids, bases, and salts.

The body's reservoir

Water is the body's most abundant substance. It performs a host of vital functions, including:
• easily forming polar covalent bonds (which permits the transport of solvents)
• acting as a lubricant in mucus and other bodily fluids
• entering into chemical reactions, such as nutrient breakdown during digestion
• enabling the body to maintain a relatively constant temperature (by both absorbing and releasing heat slowly).

I need water to stay at a constant temperature.

Recognizing ionizing

Acids, bases, and salts are *electrolytes* — compounds whose molecules consist of positively charged ions, *cations*, and negatively charged ions, *anions*, that *ionize* (separate into ions) in solution:
• *Acids* ionize into hydrogen ions (H+) and anions. In other words, acids separate into a positively charged hydrogen ion and a negatively charged anion.
• *Bases*, in contrast, ionize into hydroxide ions and cations. Bases separate into negatively charged hydroxide ions and positively charged cations.
• *Salts* form when acids react with bases. In water, salts ionize into cations and anions, but not hydrogen or hydroxide ions.

A balancing act

Body fluids must attain acid-base balance to maintain *homeostasis* (the dynamic equilibrium of the body). A solution's acidity is determined by the number of hydrogen ions it contains. The more hydrogen ions present, the more acidic the solution. Conversely, the more hydroxide ions a solution contains, the more basic, or *alkaline*, it is.

Organic compounds

Most biomolecules form *organic compounds* — compounds that contain carbon or carbon-hydrogen bonds. *Carbohydrates*, *lipids*, *proteins*, and *nucleic acids* are all examples of organic compounds.

I'm a carbohydrate. Count on me to release energy.

Carbohydrates

In the body, *carbohydrates* are sugars, starches, and glycogen.

The energy company

The main functions of carbohydrates are to release energy and store energy. There are three types of carbohydrates:

Monosaccharides, such as ribose and deoxyribose, are sugars with three to seven carbon atoms.

Disaccharides, such as lactose and maltose, contain two monosaccharides.

Polysaccharides, such as glycogen, are large carbo-hydrates with many monosaccharides.

Lipids

Lipids are water-insoluble biomolecules. The major lipids are *triglycerides*, *phospholipids*, *steroids*, *lipoproteins*, and *eicosanoids*.

To insulate and protect

Triglycerides are the most abundant lipid in both food and the body. These lipids are neutral fats that insulate and protect. They also serve as the body's most concentrated energy source. Triglycerides contain three molecules of a fatty acid chemically joined to one molecule of glycerol.

Bars on the cell

Phospholipids are the major structural components of cell membranes and consist of one molecule of glycerol, two molecules of a fatty acid, and a phosphate group.

No fat in cholesterol?

Steroids are simple lipids with no fatty acids in their molecules. They fall into four main categories, each of which performs different functions:
• *Bile salts* emulsify fats during digestion and aid absorption of the fat-soluble vitamins (vitamins A, D, E, and K).
• *Hormones* are chemical substances that have a specific effect on other cells.
• *Cholesterol*, a part of animal cell membranes, is needed to form all other steroids.
• *Vitamin D* helps regulate the body's calcium concentration.

Porters and other hardworking lipids

Lipoproteins help transport lipids to various parts of the body. *Eicosanoids* include *prostaglandins*, which, among other functions, modify hormone responses, promote the inflammatory response, and open the airways, and *leukotrienes*, which also play a part in allergic and inflammatory responses.

> **Memory jogger**
>
> To recall the distinction between the three types of carbohydrates, remember the prefixes:
> • **Mono-** means one.
> • **Di-** means two; therefore, *disaccharides* contain two monosaccharides.
> • **Poly-** means many, so you can expect that *polysaccharides* contain many monosaccharides.

Bile salts aid absorption of us fat-soluble vitamins.

Proteins

Proteins are the most abundant organic compound in the body. They're composed of building blocks called *amino acids*. Amino acids are linked together by *peptide bonds* — chemical bonds that join the carboxyl group of one amino acid to the amino group of another.

Building up the blocks

Many amino acids linked together form a *polypeptide*. One or more polypeptides form a protein. The sequence of amino acids in a protein's polypeptide chain dictates its shape. A protein's shape determines which of its many functions it performs:
- providing structure and protection
- promoting muscle contraction
- transporting various substances
- regulating processes
- serving as an enzyme (the largest group of proteins, which act as catalysts for crucial chemical reactions).

I'm a protein. I'm built from blocks of amino acids that form polypeptides.

Nucleic acids

The nucleic acids DNA and RNA are composed of nitrogenous bases, sugars, and phosphate groups. The primary hereditary molecule, DNA, contains two long chains of deoxyribonucleotides, which coil into a double-helix shape.

Holding it together

Deoxyribose and phosphate units alternate in the "backbone" of the chains. Holding the two chains together are base pairs of adenine-thymine and guanine-cytosine.

RNA and its special function

Unlike DNA, RNA has a single-chain structure. It contains ribose instead of deoxyribose and replaces the base thymine with uracil. RNA transmits genetic information from the cell nucleus to the cytoplasm. In the cytoplasm, it guides protein synthesis from amino acids.

Quick quiz

1. The three most plentiful chemical elements in the human body are:
    A.   phosphorous, hydrogen, and oxygen.
    B.   carbon, oxygen, and silicon.
    C.   oxygen, carbon, and hydrogen.
    D.   oxygen, carbon, and nitrogen.

Answer: C. There are 22 chemical elements in the human body. Oxygen (65%), carbon (18.5%), and hydrogen (9.5%) are the three most plentiful.

2. Protons are closely packed particles in the atom's nucleus that have:
    A.   a positive charge.
    B.   a negative charge.
    C.   a neutral charge.
    D.   a mixed charge.

Answer: A. Protons are positively charged particles in the atom's nucleus.

3. An example of an organic compound is:
    A.   water.
    B.   an electrolyte.
    C.   a protein.
    D.   an acid.

Answer: C. Organic compounds are compounds that contain carbon. Examples include carbohydrates, lipids, proteins, and nucleic acids.

Scoring

☆☆☆   If you answered all three questions correctly, congratulations. You and this chapter have achieved homeostasis.

☆☆   If you answered two questions correctly, excellent. You and this chapter go together as neatly as amino acids forming a polypeptide chain.

☆   If you answered only one question correctly, no worries. Get yourself organized and then go back and review the chapter.

Integumentary system

Just the facts

In this chapter, you'll learn:

♦ basic functions of the skin

♦ skin layers and their components

♦ the appendages (hair, nails, and glands) of the integumentary system.

A look at the integumentary system

The integumentary system is the largest body system and includes the skin, or *integument*, and its appendages (the hair, nails, and certain glands).

Not just another pretty face

The integumentary system performs many vital functions, including:
- protection of inner body structures
- sensory perception
- regulation of body temperature
- excretion of some body fluids.

The skin serves as the body's primary defense mechanism, protecting the body from invaders.

Protection

The skin maintains the integrity of the body surface by migration and shedding. It can repair surface wounds by intensifying normal cell replacement mechanisms. The skin's top layer, known as the *epidermis*, protects the body against noxious chemicals and invasion from bacteria and microorganisms.

Langerhans' cells to the rescue

Langerhans' cells are specialized cells within the epidermis. They enhance the body's immune response by helping lymphocytes process antigens entering the skin.

The skin's own sun block

Melanocytes, another type of skin cell, protect the skin by producing the brown pigment *melanin*, which helps filter ultraviolet light (irradiation). Exposure to ultraviolet light can stimulate melanin production.

I'm a melanocyte. I protect the body from ultraviolet light.

Sensory perception

Sensory nerve fibers originate in the nerve roots along the spine and supply sensation to specific areas of the skin known as *dermatomes*.

Just sensational

These nerve fibers transmit various sensations, such as temperature, touch, pressure, pain, and itching, from the skin to the central nervous system. Autonomic nerve fibers carry impulses to smooth muscle in the walls of the skin's blood vessels, to the muscles around the hair roots, and to the sweat glands.

Body temperature regulation

Abundant nerves, blood vessels, and eccrine glands within the skin's deeper layer, the *dermis*, help control body temperature (thermoregulation).

Warming up...

When the skin is exposed to cold or internal body temperature falls, blood vessels constrict, decreasing blood flow and thereby conserving body heat.

...and cooling down

If the skin becomes too hot or internal body temperature rises, small arteries within the skin dilate, increasing blood flow, which in turn reduces body heat. (See *The skin's role in thermoregulation.*)

Now I get it!

The skin's role in thermoregulation

Abundant nerves, blood vessels, and eccrine glands within the skin's deeper layer aid thermoregulation (control of body temperature). The first part of the flow chart shows how the body conserves body heat. The second part of the flow chart shows how the body reduces body heat. Here's how the skin does its job.

It's time to warm up

The skin becomes exposed to cold or internal body temperature falls.

Blood vessels constrict in response to stimuli from the autonomic nervous system.

Blood flow decreases through the skin and body heat is conserved.

Now let's cool things off

The skin becomes too hot or internal body temperature rises.

Small arteries in the second skin layer dilate (expand).

Increased blood flow reduces body heat. If this doesn't lower temperature, the eccrine glands act to increase sweat production, and evaporation cools the skin.

Excretion

The skin is also an excretory organ. The sweat glands excrete sweat, which contains water, electrolytes, urea, and lactic acid.

Water works

While it eliminates body wastes through its more than two million pores, the skin also prevents body fluids from escaping. Here, the skin is again protecting the body by preventing dehydration caused by loss of internal body fluids—as well as maintaining these levels by regulating the content and volume of sweat. It also keeps unwanted fluids in the environment from entering the body.

Skin layers

Two distinct layers of skin, the *epidermis* and *dermis*, lie above a third layer of *subcutaneous tissue*—sometimes called the *hypodermis*. (See *A close look at skin*.)

Epidermis

The *epidermis* is the outermost layer and varies in thickness from less than 0.1 mm on the eyelids to more than 1 mm on the palms and soles.

The ins and outs (and in betweens)

The epidermis is composed of avascular, stratified, squamous (scaly or platelike) epithelial tissue and is divided into five distinct layers. Each layer is named for its structure or function:

• The *stratum corneum* is the outermost layer and consists of tightly arranged layers of cellular membranes and keratin.

• The *stratum lucidum*, or clear layer, blocks water penetration or loss. It may be missing in some thin skin.

• The *stratum granulosum*, or granular layer, is responsible for keratin formation and, like the stratum lucidum, may be missing in some thin skin.

• The *stratum spinosum*, or spiny layer, also helps with keratin formation and is rich in ribonucleic acid.

• The *stratum basale*, or the basal layer, is the innermost layer and produces new cells to replace the superficial keratinized cells that are continuously shed or worn away.

Zoom in

A close look at skin

Major components of skin include the epidermis, dermis, and epidermal appendages.

Epidermis

Dermis

Subcutaneous tissue

Stratum corneum

Stratum basale

Papillary dermis

Sebaceous gland

Reticular dermis

Hair follicle

Eccrine sweat gland

Hair papilla

Nerve

Blood vessel

Dermis

The *dermis*, also called the *corium*, is the skin's second layer. It's an elastic system that contains and supports blood vessels, lymphatic vessels, nerves, and the epidermal appendages.

What's in the matrix?

Most of the dermis is made up of extracellular material called *matrix*. Matrix contains:
- *collagen*, a protein that gives strength to the dermis
- *elastin*, which makes the skin pliable
- *reticular fibers* that bind the collagen and elastin fibers together.

Memory jogger

You can keep straight which skin layer is which by remembering that the prefix **epi-** means "upon." Therefore, the **epi**dermis is upon, or on top of, the dermis.

The myth of fingerprints

The dermis itself has two layers:
• The *papillary dermis* has fingerlike projections, *papillae*, that connect the dermis to the epidermis. It contains characteristic ridges that on the fingers are known as fingerprints. These ridges also help the fingers and toes in gripping surfaces.
• The *reticular dermis* covers a layer of subcutaneous tissue, insulating the body to conserve heat. It also provides energy and serves as a mechanical shock absorber.

Epidermal appendages

Numerous epidermal appendages occur throughout the skin. They include the hair, nails, sebaceous glands, and sweat glands. (See *Skin, hair, and nail changes with aging.*)

Hair

Hairs are long, slender shafts composed of keratin. At the expanded lower end of each hair is a bulb or root. On its undersurface, the root is indented by a *hair papilla*, a cluster of connective tissue and blood vessels.

It will literally make your hair stand on end

Each hair lies within an epithelium-lined sheath called a *hair follicle*. A bundle of smooth-muscle fibers, *arrector pili*, extends through the dermis to attach to the base of the follicle. When these muscles contract, hair stands on end. Hair follicles also have a rich blood and nerve supply.

When arrector pili muscles contract, hair stands on end.

Nails

The *nails* are situated over the distal surface of the end of each finger and toe. Nails are composed of a specialized type of keratin.

On a bed of nails

The *nail plate*, surrounded on three sides by the nail folds, or *cuticles*, lies on the nail bed. The nail plate is

Senior moment

Skin, hair, and nail changes with aging

In the integumentary system, age-related changes can involve the skin, hair, and nails.

The skinny

As people age, their skin changes. For example, they may notice lines around their eyes (crow's feet), mouth, and nose. These lines result from subcutaneous fat loss, dermal thinning, decreasing collagen and elastin, and a 50% decline in cell replacement. Women's skin shows signs of aging about 10 years earlier than men's because it's thinner and drier.

Because of the decreased rate of skin cell replacement, wounds may heal more slowly and be prone to infection in older people. In very old people, skin loses its elasticity and may seem almost transparent. The supraclavicular and axillary regions, knuckles, and hand tendons and vessels become more prominent, as do the fat pads over bony prominences.

Other changes include the drying of mucous membranes (caused by decreased sweat gland output and number of active sweat glands). This decrease in size, number, and function of sweat glands, combined with a loss of subcutaneous fat, makes it more difficult to regulate body temperature.

Melanocyte production also decreases as a person ages; however, melanocytes often proliferate in localized areas, causing brown spots (senile lentigo). This typically occurs in areas regularly exposed to the sun. Other common skin conditions in older people include senile keratosis (dry, harsh skin) and senile angioma (a benign tumor of dilated blood vessels caused by weakened capillary walls).

Hairy situation

Hair changes also occur with aging. Hair pigment decreases and hair may turn gray or white. This loss of pigment makes hair thinner; by age 70, it's baby fine again. Hormonal changes cause pubic hair loss. At the same time, facial hair commonly increases in postmenopausal women and decreases in aging men.

Nailed down

Aging may also alter nails. They may grow at different rates, and longitudinal ridges, flaking, brittleness, and malformations may increase. Toenails may also discolor.

formed by the nail matrix, which extends proximally for about ¼″ (0.5 cm) beneath the nail fold.

Landing on the lunula

The distal portion of the matrix shows through the nail as a pale crescent-moon-shaped area. This is called the *lunula*. The translucent nail plate distal to the lunula exposes the nail bed. The vascular bed imparts the characteristic pink appearance under the nails. (See *A nail on a large scale*, page 56.)

Sebaceous glands

Sebaceous glands occur on all parts of the skin except the palms and soles. They're most prominent on the scalp, face, upper torso, and genitalia.

A nail on a large scale

The illustration below shows the anatomic components of a fingernail.

- Cuticle
- Nail bed
- Nail plate
- Lunula
- Matrix

A (small) miracle oil

The sebaceous glands produce *sebum*, a mixture of keratin, fat, and cellulose debris. Combined with sweat, sebum forms a moist, oily, acidic film that's mildly antibacterial and antifungal and that protects the skin surface. Sebum exits through the hair follicle opening to reach the skin surface.

Sweat glands

There are two types of sweat glands: eccrine glands and apocrine glands.

Eccrine glands

The *eccrine glands* are widely distributed throughout the body and produce an odorless, watery fluid with a sodium concentration equal to that of plasma. A duct from the coiled secretory portion passes through the dermis and epidermis, opening onto the skin surface.

Stressed out

Eccrine glands in the palms and soles secrete fluid mainly in response to emotional stress. For example, your ec-

Eccrine glands secrete fluid in response to stress.

crine glands might secrete fluid while you're taking a test. The remaining three million eccrine glands respond primarily to thermal stress, effectively regulating temperature.

Apocrine glands

The *apocrine glands* are located chiefly in the axillary (underarm) and anogenital (groin) areas. They have a coiled secretory portion that lies deeper in the dermis than that of the eccrine glands. A duct connects an apocrine gland to the upper portion of the hair follicle.

Oh no, b.o.

Apocrine glands begin to function at puberty. However, they have no known biological function. As bacteria decompose the fluids produced by these glands, body odor occurs.

Quick quiz

1. The main functions of the skin include:
   A. support, nourishment, and sensation.
   B. protection, sensory perception, and temperature regulation.
   C. fluid transport, sensory perception, and aging regulation.
   D. protection, motor response, and filtration.

Answer: B. The skin's main functions involve protection from injury, noxious chemicals, and bacterial invasion; sensory perception of touch, temperature, and pain; and regulation of body heat.

2. The outermost layer of the skin is the:
   A. epidermis.
   B. dermis.
   C. hypodermis.
   D. papillary dermis.

Answer: A. The outermost layer of the skin, composed of avascular, stratified, and squamous epithelial tissue, is the epidermis.

3. Which of the following integumentary system structures is considered an epidermal appendage?

A. Blood vessel
B. Nerve
C. Stratum basale
D. Hair

Answer: D. The appendages of the epidermis are the nails, hair, sebaceous glands, eccrine glands, and apocrine glands.

4. Sebum is a mixture of:

A. cellulose debris, fat, and keratin.
B. collagen and elastin.
C. watery fluid and sodium.
D. protein, water, and electrolytes.

Answer: A. Sebum is produced by the sebaceous glands and is a mixture of keratin, fat, and cellulose debris.

5. The sweat glands that are widely distributed throughout the body are:

A. apocrine.
B. eccrine.
C. adipose.
D. sebaceous.

Answer: B. Eccrine glands are widely distributed throughout the body and produce an odorless, watery fluid.

Scoring

☆☆☆   If you answered all five questions correctly, amazing! You've got the integumentary system covered.

☆☆   If you answered four questions correctly, awesome. You're scratching beneath the surface of this body system.

☆   If you answered fewer than four questions correctly, no sweat. There are still thirteen more quick quizzes to go!

Musculoskeletal system

Just the facts

In this chapter, you'll learn:

♦ major muscles and bones of the body

♦ types of muscle tissue and their functions

♦ types of bones and their functions

♦ the roles of tendons, ligaments, cartilage, joints, and bursae in body movement and structure.

A look at the musculoskeletal system

The musculoskeletal system consists of muscles, tendons, ligaments, bones, cartilage, joints, and bursae. These structures give the human body its shape and ability to move.

How the body moves

The various parts of the musculoskeletal system work with the nervous system to produce voluntary movements. Muscles contract when stimulated by impulses from the nervous system.

Using the force

During contraction, the muscle shortens, pulling on the bones to which it's attached. Force is applied to the tendon; then one bone is pulled toward, moved away from, or rotated around a second bone, depending on the type of muscle that has contracted. Most movement involves groups of muscles rather than one muscle.

Structures of the musculoskeletal system work together to provide support and produce movement.

Muscles

There are three major types of muscle in the human body. They're classified by the tissue they contain:

☝ *cardiac* (heart) muscle, which is made up of a specialized type of striated tissue

✌ *smooth* (involuntary) muscle, which contains smooth-muscle tissue

🤟 *skeletal* (voluntary and reflex) muscle, which consists of striated tissue.

The attached type

This chapter discusses only skeletal muscle — the type attached to bone. The human body has about 600 skeletal muscles. (See *Viewing the major skeletal muscles.*)

Muscle functions

Skeletal muscles move body parts or the body as a whole. They're responsible for both voluntary and reflex movements. Skeletal muscles also maintain posture and generate body heat.

Muscle structure

Skeletal muscle is composed of large, long cells called *muscle fibers*. Each fiber has many nuclei and a series of increasingly smaller internal fibrous structures. (See *Muscle structure up close*, page 62.)

Outside in

The structures of a muscle fiber, working from the cell's exterior to its interior, are:
• *endomysium* — a sheath of fibrous connective tissue that surrounds the exterior of the fiber
• *sarcolemma* — the plasma membrane of the cell that lies beneath the endomysium and just above the cell's nucleus
• *sarcoplasm* — the muscle cell's cytoplasm, which is contained within the sarcolemma

Body shop

Viewing the major skeletal muscles

This illustration shows anterior and posterior views of some of the major muscles.

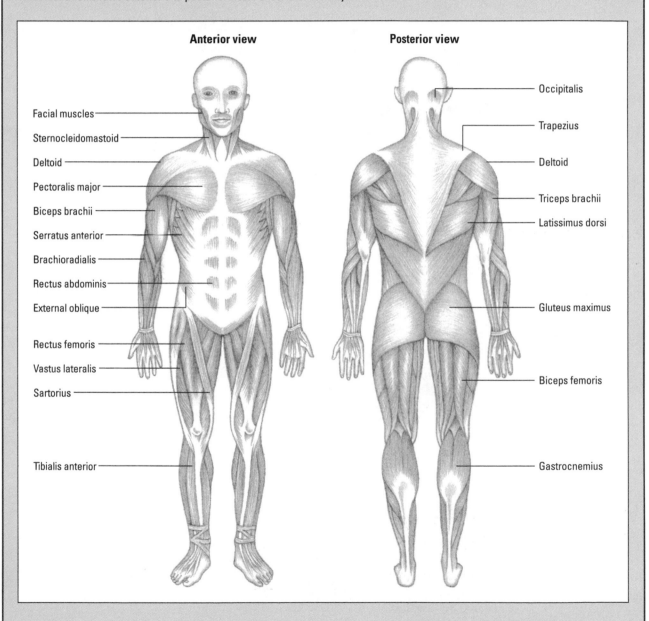

Anterior view

Facial muscles
Sternocleidomastoid
Deltoid
Pectoralis major
Biceps brachii
Serratus anterior
Brachioradialis
Rectus abdominis
External oblique
Rectus femoris
Vastus lateralis
Sartorius
Tibialis anterior

Posterior view

Occipitalis
Trapezius
Deltoid
Triceps brachii
Latissimus dorsi
Gluteus maximus
Biceps femoris
Gastrocnemius

Zoom in

Muscle structure up close

Skeletal muscle contains cell groups called *muscle fibers.* The illustration below shows the muscle and its fibers.

In a bind

The *perimysium* — a sheath of connective tissue — binds muscle fibers together into a fasciculus. The *epimysium* binds the fasciculi (bundles of muscle fibers) together; beyond the muscle, it becomes a tendon.

Surrounded

A sarcolemma (plasma membrane) surrounds each muscle fiber. Tiny myofibrils within the muscle fibers contain even finer fibers called *myosin* (thick filaments) and *actin* (thin filaments).

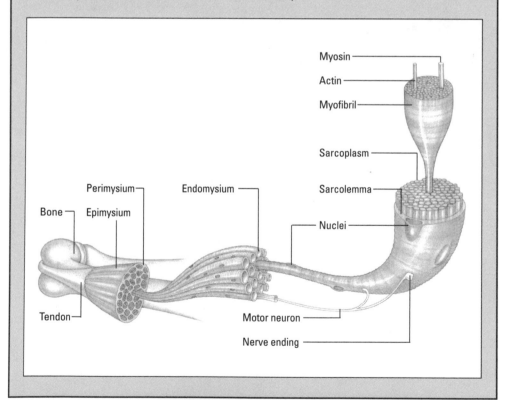

- *myofibrils* — tiny, threadlike structures that run the fiber's length and make up the bulk of the fiber
- *myosin* (thick filaments) and *actin* (thin filaments) — still finer fibers within the myofibrils; there are about 1,500 myosin and about 3,000 actin.

Sarcomeres end to end

Myosin and actin are contained within compartments called *sarcomeres*. Sarcomeres are the functional units of skeletal muscle. During muscle contraction, myosin and actin slide over each other, reducing sarcomere length.

Zebra stripes

The sarcomere compartments of all the myofibrils in a single fiber are aligned. When a muscle fiber is viewed microscopically, transverse (at right angles to the long axis) stripes, called *striations* (or Z-lines), appear along the length of the fiber.

A bundle of bundles

A fibrous sheath of connective tissue, called the *perimysium*, binds muscle fibers into a bundle, or *fasciculus*. A stronger sheath, the *epimysium*, binds all of the fasciculi together to form the entire muscle. Extending beyond the muscle, the epimysium becomes a tendon.

Muscle attachment

Most skeletal muscles are attached to bones, either directly or indirectly.

The direct approach

In a direct attachment, the epimysium of the muscle fuses to the *periosteum*, the fibrous membrane covering the bone.

Being indirect

In an indirect attachment (most common), the epimysium extends past the muscle as a tendon, or *aponeurosis*, and attaches to the bone.

Contraction

During contraction, one of the bones to which the muscle is attached stays relatively stationary while the other is pulled in toward the stationary one.

Origin and insertion

The point where the muscle attaches to the stationary or less movable bone is called the *origin;* the point where it attaches to the more movable bone is called the *inser-*

When I contract my muscles to lift this cup, one bone stays stationary. The other bone is pulled toward the stationary one.

tion. The origin usually lies on the proximal end of the bone. The insertion site is on the distal end.

Muscle growth

Muscle develops when existing muscle fibers hypertrophy. Muscle strength and size differ among individuals because of such factors as exercise, nutrition, gender, age, and genetic constitution. Changes in nutrition or exercise cause muscle strength and size to vary in an individual. (See *Musculoskeletal changes with aging.*)

Factors such as genetic constitution and exercise cause muscle strength and size to differ among individuals.

Muscle movements

Skeletal muscle can permit several types of movement. A muscle's functional name comes from the type of movement it permits. For example, a flexor muscle permits bending *(flexion)*; an adductor muscle permits movement toward a body axis *(adduction)*; and a circumductor muscle allows a circular movement *(circumduction).* (See *Basics of body movement.*)

Senior moment

Musculoskeletal changes with aging

As an individual ages, the most apparent musculoskeletal change is usually decreasing height. This occurs because exaggerated spinal curvature and narrowed intervertebral spaces cause the trunk to shorten and the arms to appear relatively long.

Other musculoskeletal changes that occur with aging include decreased muscle mass, which may result in muscle weakness, and decreased bone density. In addition, collagen formation declines, which causes joints and supporting structures to lose resilience and elasticity. Synovial fluid also becomes more viscous and synovial membranes become more fibrotic, making joints stiff.

Aging may also make tandem walking difficult. Usually, elderly people walk with shorter steps and wider leg stances for better balance and stability.

Body shop

Basics of body movement

Basic muscle movement is best demonstrated in the diarthrodial joints, which allow 13 angular and circular movements:
- The shoulder demonstrates circumduction.
- The elbow demonstrates flexion and extension.
- The hip demonstrates internal and external rotation.
- The arm demonstrates abduction and adduction.
- The hand demonstrates supination and pronation.
- The jaw demonstrates retraction and protraction.
- The foot demonstrates eversion and inversion.

Retraction and protraction
Moving backward and forward

Extension
Straightening, increasing the joint angle

Flexion
Bending, decreasing the joint angle

Abduction
Moving away from the midline

Adduction
Moving toward the midline

Circumduction
Moving in a circular manner

Pronation
Turning downward

Supination
Turning upward

Internal rotation
Turning toward the midline

External rotation
Turning away from the midline

Eversion
Turning outward

Inversion
Turning inward

Muscles of the axial skeleton

The muscles of the axial skeleton are essential for respiration, speech, facial expression, posture, and chewing. They include:
- muscles of the face, tongue, and neck
- muscles of mastication
- muscles of the vertebral column situated along the spine.

Muscles of the appendicular skeleton

The appendicular skeleton includes the muscles of the:
- shoulder
- abdominopelvic cavity
- upper and lower extremities.
    Muscles of the upper extremities are classified according to the bones they move. Those that move the arm are further categorized into those with an origin on the axial skeleton and those with an origin on the scapula.

Tendons and ligaments

Tendons are bands of fibrous connective tissue that attach muscles to the periosteum, the fibrous covering of the bone. Tendons enable bones to move when skeletal muscles contract.
    Ligaments are dense, strong, flexible bands of fibrous connective tissue that bind bones to other bones.

Bones

The human skeleton contains 206 bones: 80 form the *axial skeleton* — called *axial* because it lies along the central line, or axis, of the body — and 126 form the *appendicular skeleton* — relating to the limbs, or appendages, of the body. (See *Viewing the major bones.*)

Access the axis

Bones of the axial skeleton include:
- facial and cranial bones
- hyoid bone

Body shop

Viewing the major bones

The illustrations below show the major bones and bone groups in the body.

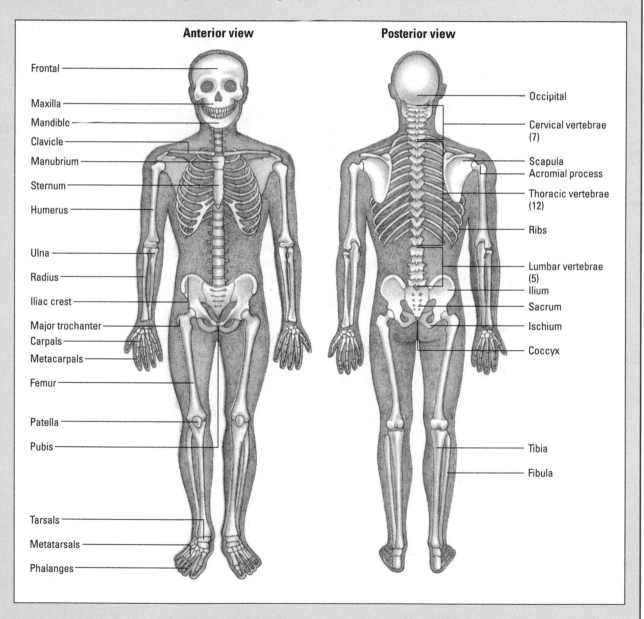

Anterior view

Frontal
Maxilla
Mandible
Clavicle
Manubrium
Sternum
Humerus
Ulna
Radius
Iliac crest
Major trochanter
Carpals
Metacarpals
Femur
Patella
Pubis
Tarsals
Metatarsals
Phalanges

Posterior view

Occipital
Cervical vertebrae (7)
Scapula
Acromial process
Thoracic vertebrae (12)
Ribs
Lumbar vertebrae (5)
Ilium
Sacrum
Ischium
Coccyx
Tibia
Fibula

- vertebrae
- ribs and sternum.

Appendages to the axis

Bones of the appendicular skeleton include:
- clavicle
- scapula
- humerus, radius, ulna, carpals, metacarpals, and phalanges
- pelvic bones
- femur, patella, fibula, tibia, tarsals, metatarsals, and phalanges.

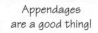

Appendages are a good thing!

You think you're humerus, don't you?

Bone classification

Bones are typically classified by shape. Thus, bones may be classified as:
- long (such as the humerus, radius, femur, and tibia) (see *Viewing a long bone*)
- short (such as the carpals and tarsals)
- flat (such as the scapula, ribs, and skull)
- irregular (such as the vertebrae and mandible)
- sesamoid, meaning "resembling a sesame seed" (such as the patella).

Bone functions

Bones perform various anatomic (mechanical) and physiologic functions. They:
- protect internal tissues and organs
- stabilize and support the body
- provide a surface for muscle, ligament, and tendon attachment
- move through "lever" action when contracted
- produce red blood cells in the bone marrow (*hematopoiesis*)
- store mineral salts (such as 99% of the body's calcium).

I support and stabilize the body.

Zoom in

Viewing a long bone

The main parts of a long bone, shown below, are the *diaphysis* (shaft) and the *epiphyses* (ends). Periosteum surrounds the diaphysis; endosteum lines the medullary cavity. At the epiphyseal line, cartilage separates the epiphyses from the diaphysis.

Two types of bone tissue

Each bone consists of an outer layer of dense, smooth compact bone, which contains haversian canals, and an inner layer of spongy cancellous bone, which lacks these canals.

Cancellous bone

Cancellous bone consists of tiny spikes, called *trabeculae,* that interlace to form a latticework. Red marrow fills the spaces between the trabeculae of some bones. Cancellous bone fills the central regions of the epiphyses and the inner portions of short, flat, and irregular bones.

Compact bone

Compact bone is found in the diaphyses of long bones and the outer layers of short, flat, and irregular bones. Compact bone consists of layers of calcified matrix containing spaces occupied by osteocytes (bone cells). *Lamellae* (bone layers) are arranged around central canals (haversian canals). Small cavities called *lacunae,* which lie between the lamellae, contain osteocytes. Canaliculi (tiny canals) connect the lacunae, forming the structural units of the bone. Canaliculi also provide nutrients to bone tissue.

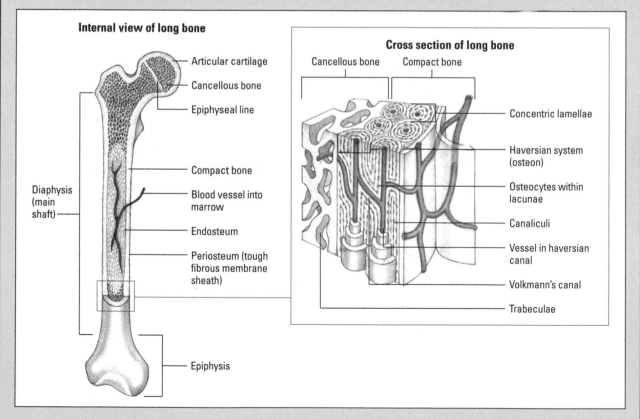

Internal view of long bone

- Articular cartilage
- Cancellous bone
- Epiphyseal line
- Compact bone
- Blood vessel into marrow
- Endosteum
- Periosteum (tough fibrous membrane sheath)

Diaphysis (main shaft)

Epiphysis

Cross section of long bone

Cancellous bone   Compact bone

- Concentric lamellae
- Haversian system (osteon)
- Osteocytes within lacunae
- Canaliculi
- Vessel in haversian canal
- Volkmann's canal
- Trabeculae

Blood supply

Blood reaches bones through three paths:

👆 *haversian canals*, minute channels that lie parallel to the axis of the bone and are passages for arterioles

✌️ *Volkmann's canals*, which contain vessels that connect one haversian canal to another and to the outer bone

🤟 *vessels* in the bone ends and within the marrow.

Bone formation

At 3 months in utero, the fetal skeleton is composed of cartilage. By about 6 months, fetal cartilage has been transformed into bony skeleton. (See *Bone growth and remodeling*.)

Ossification is hard work

After birth, some bones — most notably the carpals and tarsals — *ossify* (harden). The change results from *endochondral ossification*, a process by which *osteoblasts* (bone-forming cells) produce *osteoid* (a collagenous material that ossifies).

Bone remodeling

Two types of osteocytes, osteoblasts and osteoclasts, are responsible for *remodeling* — the continuous process whereby bone is created and destroyed.

Blast them bones

Osteoblasts deposit new bone, and *osteoclasts* increase long-bone diameter. Osteoclasts promote longitudinal bone growth by reabsorbing the previously deposited bone. This growth continues until the *epiphyseal plates* ossify during late adolescence. The epiphyseal plates are cartilage that separate the *diaphysis*, or shaft of a bone, from the *epiphysis*, or end of a bone.

Memory jogger

To remember the function of osteocytes (bone remodeling), remember that they do all the "cyte" (site) work like anyone in construction.

Zoom in

Bone growth and remodeling

The ossification of cartilage into bone, or *osteogenesis,* begins at about the ninth week of fetal development. The diaphyses of long bones are formed by birth, and the epiphyses begin to ossify at about that time. Below are the stages of bone growth and remodeling of the epiphyses of a long bone.

Creation of an ossification center

At about the ninth month, an ossification center develops in the epiphysis. Some cartilage cells enlarge and stimulate ossification of surrounding cells. The enlarged cells die, leaving small cavities. New cartilage continues to develop.

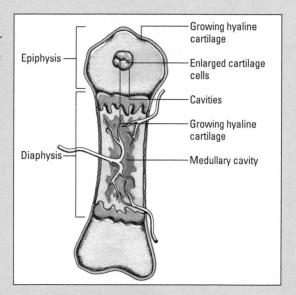

Growing hyaline cartilage

Epiphysis

Enlarged cartilage cells

Cavities

Growing hyaline cartilage

Diaphysis

Medullary cavity

Osteoblasts form bone

Osteoblasts begin to form bone on the remaining cartilage, creating the trabeculae network of cancellous bone. Cartilage continues to form on the outer surfaces of the epiphysis and along the upper surface of the epiphyseal plate.

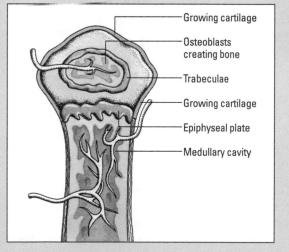

Growing cartilage

Osteoblasts creating bone

Trabeculae

Growing cartilage

Epiphyseal plate

Medullary cavity

(continued)

Bone growth and remodeling *(continued)*

Bone length grows

Cartilage is replaced by compact bone near the outer surfaces of the epiphysis. Only cartilage cells on the upper surface of the epiphyseal plate continue to multiply rapidly, pushing the epiphysis away from the diaphysis. This new cartilage ossifies, creating trabeculae on the medullary side of the epiphyseal plate.

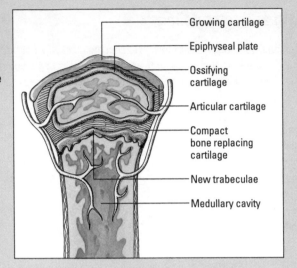

Growing cartilage

Epiphyseal plate

Ossifying cartilage

Articular cartilage

Compact bone replacing cartilage

New trabeculae

Medullary cavity

Remodeling

Osteoclasts produce enzymes and acids that reduce trabeculae created by the epiphyseal plate, thus enlarging the medullary cavity. In the epiphysis, osteoclasts reduce bone, making its calcium available for new osteoblasts that give the epiphysis its adult shape and proportion. In young adults, the epiphyseal plate completely ossifies (closes) and becomes the epiphyseal line; longitudinal growth of bone then ceases.

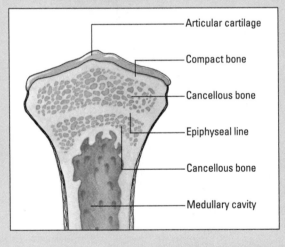

Articular cartilage

Compact bone

Cancellous bone

Epiphyseal line

Cancellous bone

Medullary cavity

Bone density decreases after age 30 in women and after age 45 in men.

Cartilage

Cartilage is a dense connective tissue that consists of fibers embedded in a strong, gel-like substance. Unlike rigid bone, cartilage has the flexibility of firm plastic.

Cartilage supports and shapes various structures, such as the auditory canal and the intervertebral disks.

It also cushions and absorbs shock, preventing direct transmission to the bone. Cartilage has no blood supply or innervation.

There are three types of cartilage:

 hyaline

 fibrous

 elastic.

Common connector

Hyaline cartilage is the most common type of cartilage. It covers the articular bone surfaces (where one or more bones meet at a joint). It also connects the ribs to the sternum and appears in the trachea, bronchi, and nasal septum.

The strong, rigid type

Fibrous cartilage forms the symphysis pubis and the intervertebral disks. This type of cartilage is composed of small quantities of matrix and abundant fibrous elements. It's strong and rigid.

Staying flexible

Elastic cartilage is located in the auditory canal, external ear, and epiglottis. Large numbers of elastic fibers give this type of cartilage elasticity and resiliency.

Joints

Joints (articulations) are points of contact between two bones that hold the bones together. Many joints also allow flexibility and movement.

It's the joint

Joints can be classified by function (extent of movement) or by structure (what they're made of). The body has three major types of joints classified by function and three major types classified by structure.

Hey, I know a joint where we can get together.

Functional classification

By function, a joint may be classified as:

- *synarthrosis* (immovable)
- *amphiarthrosis* (slightly movable)
- *diarthrosis* (freely movable).

Structural classification

By structure, a joint may be classified as:

- fibrous
- cartilaginous
- synovial.

Fibrous joints

In *fibrous joints*, the articular surfaces of the two bones are bound closely by fibrous connective tissue, and little movement is possible. Fibrous joints include *sutures*, *syndesmoses* (such as the radioulnar joints), and *gomphoses* (such as the dental alveolar joint).

Cartilaginous joints

In *cartilaginous joints* (also called amphiarthroses), cartilage connects one bone to another. Cartilaginous joints allow slight movement. They occur as:
- *synchondroses*, which are typically temporary joints in which the intervening hyaline cartilage converts to bone by adulthood — for example, the epiphyseal plates of long bones
- *symphyses*, which are joints with an intervening pad of fibrocartilage — for example, the symphysis pubis.

Synovial joints

The contiguous bony surfaces in the *synovial joints* are separated by a viscous, lubricating fluid — the *synovia* — and by cartilage. They're joined by ligaments lined with a synovia-producing membrane. Freely movable, synovial joints include most joints of the arms and legs.

Synovial joints are freely movable and include most joints of the arms and legs.

Other features of synovial joints include:
- a *joint cavity* — a potential space that separates the articulating surfaces of the two bones
- an *articular capsule* — a saclike envelope with an outer layer that's lined with a vascular synovial membrane
- *reinforcing ligaments* — fibrous tissue that connects bones within the joint and reinforces the joint capsule.

Based on their structure and the type of movement they allow, synovial joints fall into various subdivisions — gliding, hinge, pivot, condylar, saddle, and ball-and-socket.

Let it glide

Gliding joints have flat or slightly curved articular surfaces and allow gliding movements. However, because they're bound by ligaments, they may not allow movement in all directions. Examples of gliding joints are the intertarsal and intercarpal joints of the hands and feet.

Here's a hinge

In *hinge joints*, a convex portion of one bone fits into a concave portion of another. The movement of a hinge joint resembles that of a metal hinge and is limited to flexion and extension. Hinge joints include the elbow and knee.

Apply your muscles and the lever moves. Wheeeee!

Bones are like levers; joints are like fulcrums.

"Pivotal" joints

A rounded portion of one bone in a *pivot joint* fits into a groove in another bone. Pivot joints allow only uniaxial rotation of the first bone around the second. An example of a pivot joint is the head of the radius, which rotates within a groove of the ulna.

Give condylar joints a hand

In *condylar joints*, an oval surface of one bone fits into a concavity in another bone. Condylar joints allow flexion, extension, abduction, adduction, and circumduction. Examples include the radiocarpal and metacarpophalangeal joints of the hand.

Saddle up

Saddle joints resemble condylar joints but allow greater freedom of movement. The only saddle joints in the body are the carpometacarpal joints of the thumb.

Ball-and-socket: These joints are hip

The *ball-and-socket joint* gets its name from the way its bones connect: The spherical head of one bone fits into a concave "socket" of another bone. The body's only ball-and-socket joints are the shoulder and hip joints.

Bursae

Bursae are small synovial fluid sacs that are located at friction points around joints between tendons, ligaments, and bones.

Stress reducers

Bursae act as cushions to decrease stress on adjacent structures. Examples of bursae include the subacromial bursa (located in the shoulder) and the prepatellar bursa (located in the knee).

The ball-and-socket is the hippest joint around. It allows more freedom of movement than any other synovial joint.

Quick quiz

1. Which muscle type is considered voluntary (contraction is controlled at will)?
    A.   Cardiac
    B.   Smooth
    C.   Skeletal
    D.   Epimysium

Answer: C. Skeletal muscle is voluntary, meaning it can be moved at will. The musculoskeletal system consists mostly of skeletal muscle.

2. Which of the following statements about cartilage is true?
    A.   It receives a generous blood supply.
    B.   It protects body structures.
    C.   It's completely flexible.
    D.   It cushions and absorbs shock.

Answer: D. Cartilage is responsible for supporting, cushioning, and shaping body structures. Types of cartilage include fibrous, hyaline, and elastic.

3. The type of joint that permits free movement is classified as:
    A.   synarthrosis.
    B.   cartilaginous.
    C.   diarthrosis.
    D.   fibrous.

Answer: C. Diarthroses include the ankles, wrists, knees, hips, and shoulders. These joints permit free movement.

4. The carpometacarpal joints of the thumb are classified as:
    A.   pivot joints.
    B.   saddle joints.
    C.   hinge joints.
    D.   gliding joints.

Answer: B. Saddle joints are similar to condylar joints. The only saddle joints in the body are the carpometacarpal joints of the thumbs.

Scoring

☆☆☆　If you answered all four questions correctly, outstanding! You've flexed your mental muscles and are ready to tackle the next system.

☆☆　If you answered three questions correctly, splendid! You've got the bare bones of this system down pat.

☆　If you answered fewer than three questions correctly, that's okay. Let's take our osteocytes and blast into the next chapter.

Nervous system

Just the facts

In this chapter, you'll learn:

♦ structures of the nervous system

♦ functions of the nervous system

♦ special sense organs and their functions.

A look at the nervous system

The nervous system coordinates all body functions, enabling a person to adapt to changes in internal and external environments. It has two main types of cells:
• neurons, the conducting cells
• neuroglia, the supportive cells.

Neuron: The basic unit

The *neuron* is the basic unit of the nervous system. This highly specialized conductor cell receives and transmits electrochemical nerve impulses. Delicate, threadlike nerve fibers called *axons* and *dendrites* extend from the central cell body and transmit signals. In a typical neuron, one axon and many dendrites extend from the cell body. (See *Parts of a neuron*, page 80.)

Axons

Axons conduct nerve impulses away from cell bodies. A typical axon has terminal branches and is wrapped in a white, fatty, segmented covering called a *myelin sheath*. The myelin sheath is produced by *Schwann cells* — phagocytic cells separated by gaps called *nodes of Ranvier.*

I'm a neuron, the fundamental unit of the nervous system.

Zoom in

Parts of a neuron

A typical neuron, like the one shown here, has one axon and many dendrites. A myelin sheath encloses the axon.

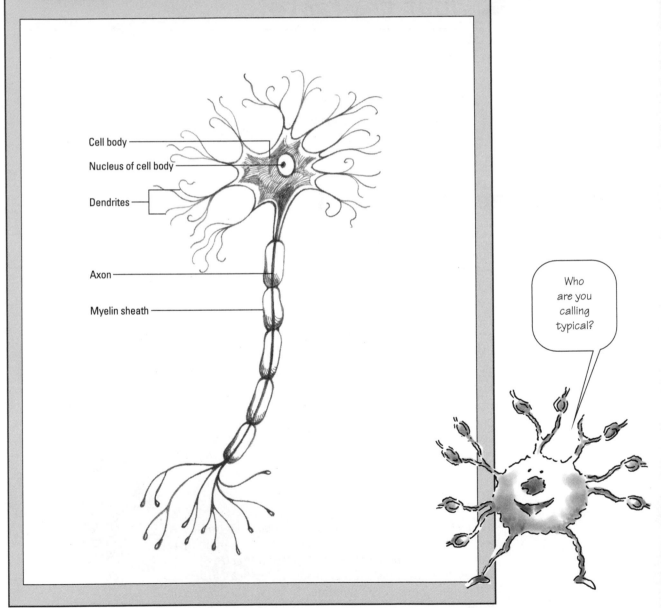

Cell body

Nucleus of cell body

Dendrites

Axon

Myelin sheath

Who are you calling typical?

Dendrites

Dendrites are short, thick, diffusely branched extensions of the cell body that receive impulses from other cells. Dendrites conduct impulses toward the cell body.

Sending the message

Neurons are responsible for *neurotransmission* — conduction of electrochemical impulses throughout the nervous system. Neuron activity may be provoked by:
• mechanical stimuli, such as touch and pressure
• thermal stimuli, such as heat and cold
• chemical stimuli, such as external chemicals or a chemical released by the body, such as histamine. (See *How neurotransmission occurs*, page 82.)

> Thermal stimuli such as heat produce neuron activity and start conduction of electrochemical impulses through the nervous system.

Neuroglia

Neuroglia (also called *glial cells*) are the supportive cells of the nervous system. They form roughly 40% of the brain's bulk.

Neuroglia to know

Four types of neuroglia exist:

  Astroglia, or *astrocytes*, exist throughout the nervous system. They supply nutrients to neurons and help them maintain their electrical potential. They also form part of the blood-brain barrier.

  Ependymal cells line the four small cavities in the brain, called *ventricles*, and the choroid plexuses. They help produce cerebrospinal fluid (CSF).

  Microglia are phagocytic cells that ingest and digest microorganisms and waste products from injured neurons.

  Oligodendroglia support and electrically insulate central nervous system (CNS) axons by forming protective myelin sheaths.

> Glial is derived from the Greek word for glue. Glial cells "glue" the neurons together.

Now I get it!

How neurotransmission occurs

Neurons receive and transmit stimuli by electrochemical messages. Dendrites on the neuron receive an impulse sent by other cells and conduct it toward the cell body. The axon then conducts the impulse away from the cell.

To stimulate or inhibit
When the impulse reaches the end of the axon, it stimulates synaptic vesicles in the presynaptic axon terminal. A neurotransmitter substance is then released into the synaptic cleft between neurons. This substance diffuses across the synaptic cleft and binds to special receptors on the postsynaptic membrane. This stimulates or inhibits stimulation of the postsynaptic neuron.

Central nervous system

The CNS includes the brain and the spinal cord. Encased by the bones of the skull and vertebral column, the CNS is protected by the CSF and the meninges (the dura mater, arachnoid, and pia mater).

Brain

The brain consists of the cerebrum, cerebellum, brain stem, diencephalon (thalamus and hypothalamus), limbic system, and reticular activating system.

Cerebrum

The *cerebrum* is the largest part of the brain. It houses the nerve center that controls sensory and motor activities and intelligence.

Touch of gray

The outer layer of the cerebrum, the *cerebral cortex*, consists of unmyelinated nerve fibers *(gray matter)*. The inner layer of the cerebrum consists of myelinated nerve fibers.

Steady as she goes

Within the cerebrum lies *white matter* (myelinated nerve fibers). *Basal ganglia*, which control motor coordination and steadiness, are found in white matter.

Bridging the hemispheres

The cerebrum has right and left hemispheres. A mass of nerve fibers known as the *corpus callosum* bridges the hemispheres, allowing communication between corresponding centers in each hemisphere. The rolling surface of the cerebrum is made up of *gyri* (convolutions) and *sulci* (creases or fissures).

The corpus callosum allows communication between the two hemispheres.

The four lobes

Each cerebral hemisphere is divided into four lobes, based on anatomic landmarks and functional differences. These lobes—the frontal, temporal, parietal, and occipital—are named for the cranial bones that lie over them. (See *A close look at major brain structures*.)

Cerebellum

The *cerebellum* is the brain's second largest region. It lies behind and below the cerebrum. Like the cerebrum, it has two hemispheres. It also has an outer cortex of gray matter and an inner core of white matter. The cerebellum functions to maintain muscle tone, coordinate muscle movement, and control balance.

Brain stem

The *brain stem* lies immediately below the cerebrum, just in front of the cerebellum. It continues from the cerebrum above and connects with the spinal cord below.

It all stems from the brain stem

The brain stem consists of the *midbrain, pons,* and *medulla oblongata.* It relays messages between the parts of the nervous system and has three main functions:
• It produces the vital autonomic reactions necessary for survival, such as increasing heart rate and stimulating the adrenal medulla to produce epinephrine.
• It provides pathways for nerve fibers between higher and lower neural centers.
• It serves as the origin for 10 of the 12 pairs of cranial nerves.

Thanks to the brain stem, I can communicate with the rest of the nervous system.

It goes both ways

The three parts of the brain stem provide two-way conduction between the spinal cord and brain. In addition, they perform the following functions:
• The *midbrain* is the reflex center for cranial nerves (CNs) III and IV and mediates pupillary reflexes and eye movements.
• The *pons* helps regulate respirations. It connects the cerebellum with the cerebrum and links the midbrain to the medulla oblongata. It's also the reflex center for CNs V through VIII. The pons mediates chewing, taste, saliva secretion, hearing, and equilibrium.
• The *medulla oblongata* joins the spinal cord at the level of the *foramen magnum,* an opening in the occipital portion of the skull. It influences cardiac, respiratory, and

Zoom in

A close look at major brain structures

The illustration below shows the two largest structures of the brain—the cerebrum and cerebellum. Several fissures divide the cerebrum into hemispheres and lobes:

• The *fissure of Sylvius,* or the lateral sulcus, separates the temporal lobe from the frontal and parietal lobes.

• The *fissure of Rolando,* or the central sulcus, separates the frontal lobes from the parietal lobe.

• The *parieto-occipital fissure* separates the occipital lobe from the two parietal lobes.

To each lobe, a function

Each lobe has a particular function:

• The *frontal lobe* influences personality, judgment, abstract reasoning, social behavior, language expression, and voluntary movement (in the motor portion).

• The *temporal lobe* controls hearing, language comprehension, and storage and recall of memories (although memories are stored throughout the entire brain).

• The *parietal lobe* interprets and integrates sensations, including pain, temperature, and touch. It also interprets size, shape, distance, and texture. The parietal lobe of the nondominant hemisphere is especially important for awareness of body shape.

• The *occipital lobe* functions mainly to interpret visual stimuli.

Parietal lobe

Parieto-occipital fissure

Occipital lobe

Fissure of Sylvius

Temporal lobe

Cerebellum

Sensory cortex

Motor cortex

Fissure of Rolando

Frontal lobe

I've got a charming personality, thanks to my frontal lobe.

vasomotor functions. It's the center for the vomiting, coughing, and hiccuping reflexes.

Diencephalon

The *diencephalon* is the part of the brain located between the cerebrum and the midbrain. It consists of the thalamus and hypothalamus, which lie deep in the cerebral hemispheres.

Screening calls

The *thalamus* relays all sensory stimuli (except olfactory) as they ascend to the cerebral cortex. Its functions include primitive awareness of pain, screening of incoming stimuli, and focusing of attention.

Control center

The *hypothalamus* controls or affects body temperature, appetite, water balance, pituitary secretions, emotions, and autonomic functions, including sleeping and waking cycles.

Limbic system

The *limbic system* is a primitive brain area deep within the temporal lobe. In addition to initiating basic drives (such as hunger, aggression, and emotional and sexual arousal) the limbic system screens all sensory messages traveling to the cerebral cortex.

Reticular activating system

The *reticular activating system* (RAS) is a diffuse network of hyperexcitable neurons. It fans out from the brain stem through the cerebral cortex. After screening all incoming sensory information, the RAS channels it to appropriate areas of the brain for interpretation. It functions as the arousal, or alerting, system for the cerebral cortex and is crucial in maintaining consciousness. (See *Neurologic changes with aging.*)

Oxygenating the brain

Four major arteries—two vertebral and two carotid— supply the brain with oxygenated blood.

(Text continues on page 87.)

> My thalamus acts as a relay station. Sensory impulses cross synapses in the thalamus on their way to the cerebral cortex.

Senior moment

Neurologic changes with aging

Aging affects the nervous system in many ways. For example, neurons of the central and peripheral nervous systems undergo degenerative changes. After about age 50, the number of brain cells decreases by about 1% per year. However, clinical effects usually aren't noticeable until aging advances further.

As a person ages, the hypothalamus becomes less effective at regulating body temperature. Also, the cerebral cortex undergoes a 20% neuron loss. Because nerve transmission typically slows down, elderly people may react sluggishly to external stimuli.

Incredibly Easy miniguide to anatomy: The brain

The illustrations below show the four lobes of the brain and structures of the limbic system.

> Each of my cerebral hemispheres is divided into four lobes, and each lobe is named for the cranial bones that lay over it.

Lobes of the brain

- Frontal lobe
- Parietal lobe
- Occipital lobe
- Temporal lobe
- Cerebellum

> The *limbic system* is a primitive brain area deep within the temporal lobe that initiates basic drives, such as hunger, aggression, and emotional and sexual arousal. It also screens all sensory messages traveling to the cerebral cortex.

Limbic system

- Cingulate gyrus
- Corpus callosum
- Mammillary body
- Olfactory tract
- Amygdala
- Hippocampus

Incredibly Easy miniguide to anatomy: The skeletal system

These illustrations show anterior and posterior views of some of the major bones.

I'm important. After all, bones protect internal tissues and organs, stabilize and support the body, allow motion, and provide a surface for muscle, ligament, and tendon attachment.

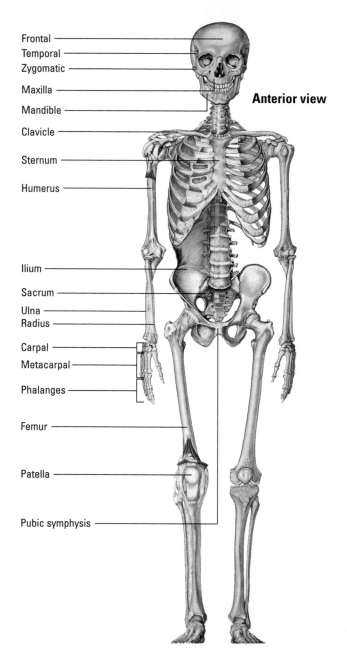

Frontal
Temporal
Zygomatic
Maxilla
Mandible
Clavicle
Sternum
Humerus
Ilium
Sacrum
Ulna
Radius
Carpal
Metacarpal
Phalanges
Femur
Patella
Pubic symphysis

Anterior view

Incredibly Easy miniguide to anatomy: The skeletal system

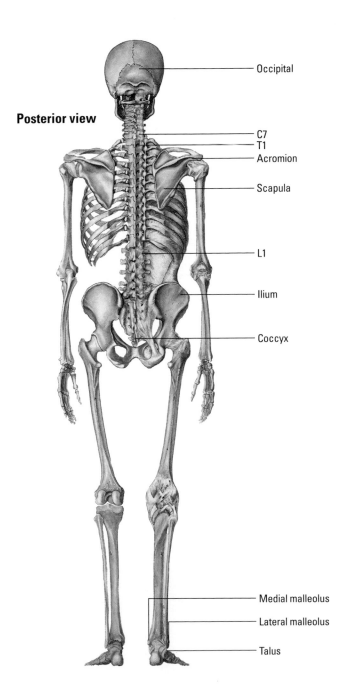

Posterior view

Occipital

C7
T1
Acromion

Scapula

L1

Ilium

Coccyx

Medial malleolus

Lateral malleolus

Talus

That's not all! Bones also produce red blood cells in the bone marrow and store mineral salts such as calcium.

Incredibly Easy miniguide to anatomy: The muscular system

These illustrations show some of the major muscles of the body.

Skeletal muscles move body parts or the body as a whole. They're used for both voluntary and reflex movements.

Anterior view

Deltoid

Pectoralis major

Rectus abdominis

Biceps brachii

Brachialis

External abdominal oblique

Flexor pollicis longus

Abductor pollicis longus

Pronator quadratus

Flexor retinaculum

Vastus intermedius

Vastus lateralis

Vastus medialis

Patellar ligament

Soleus

Tibialis anterior

Incredibly Easy miniguide to anatomy: The muscular system

Posterior view

- Occipitalis
- Trapezius
- Deltoid
- Rhomboid major
- Triceps brachii
- Brachialis
- Latissimus dorsi
- Gluteus maximus
- Biceps femoris
- Vastus lateralis
- Sartorius
- Gastrocnemius

Skeletal muscles also help maintain posture and generate body heat.

Incredibly Easy miniguide to anatomy: The heart

The heart is located beneath the sternum in the mediastinum. It rests on the superior surface of the diaphragm and lies anterior to the vertebral column.

Anterior view

Arch of aorta

Superior vena cava

Pericardial sac

Atrioventricular valve (tricuspid)

Papillary muscles

Right ventricle (opened)

Wow! I'm actually two separate pumps. My right side pumps blood to the lungs, and my left side pumps blood to the rest of the body.

Section of heart wall

Fibrous pericardium

Parietal pericardium

Pericardial cavity

Epicardium

Myocardium

Endocardium

Incredibly Easy miniguide to anatomy: The heart

The myocardium receives blood through four main coronary arteries, as shown below.

Anterior view

Aorta
Superior vena cava
Main pulmonary artery
Left atrium
Right atrium
Left ventricle
Right ventricle

Posterior view

Aorta
Superior vena cava
Pulmonary arteries
Pulmonary veins
Left atrium
Right atrium
Left ventricle
Right ventricle

Coronary arteries

Aorta
Left main coronary artery
Left circumflex artery
Right coronary artery
Left anterior descending artery

I rely on the coronary arteries and their branches for a healthy supply of oxygenated blood. Thanks guys!

ANATOMY & PHYSIOLOGY MADE
Incredibly Easy
2nd edition

Incredibly Easy miniguide to anatomy: The respiratory system

The pathways through which air travels to reach the lungs include the nasal and oral cavities, oropharynx, trachea, and bronchi. Air is warmed, filtered, moistened, and delivered to and from the gas exchange area of the lungs.

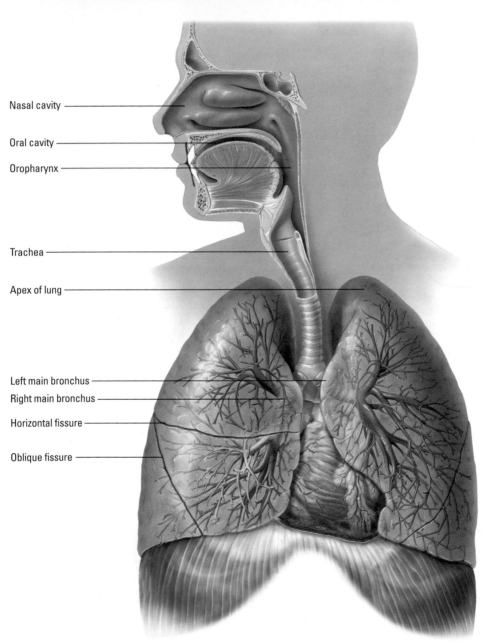

Nasal cavity

Oral cavity

Oropharynx

Trachea

Apex of lung

Left main bronchus

Right main bronchus

Horizontal fissure

Oblique fissure

Dig it. I'm at the center of the body system that maintains the exchange of oxygen and carbon dioxide.

Incredibly Easy miniguide to anatomy: The respiratory system

The respiratory unit consists of the respiratory bronchiole, alveolar duct and sac, and alveoli. Gas exchange occurs rapidly in the alveoli, in which oxygen from inhaled air diffuses into the blood and carbon dioxide diffuses from the blood into exhaled air.

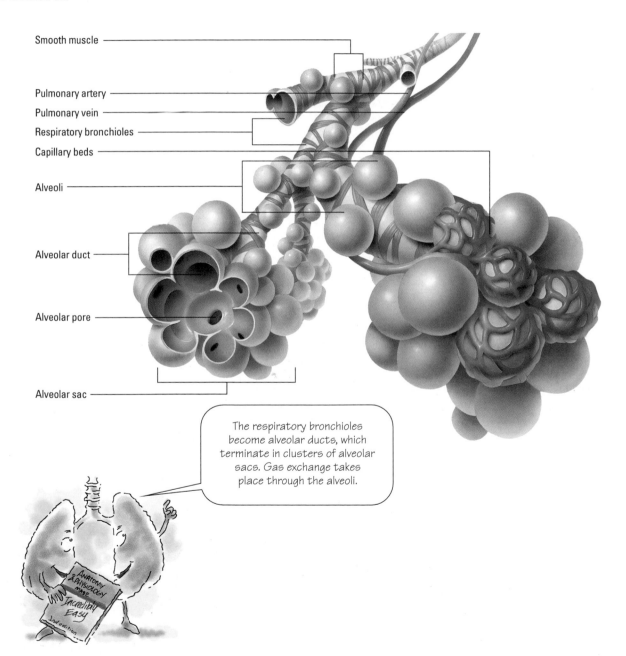

Smooth muscle

Pulmonary artery

Pulmonary vein

Respiratory bronchioles

Capillary beds

Alveoli

Alveolar duct

Alveolar pore

Alveolar sac

The respiratory bronchioles become alveolar ducts, which terminate in clusters of alveolar sacs. Gas exchange takes place through the alveoli.

Incredibly Easy miniguide to anatomy: The spinal nerves

There are 31 pairs of spinal nerves. After leaving the spinal cord, many nerves join together to form networks called *plexuses,* as this illustration shows.

Cervical plexus

Brachial plexus

Lumbar plexus

Sacral plexus

Cervical nerves (C1 to C8)

Thoracic nerves (T1 to T12)

Lumbar nerves (L1 to L5)

Sacral nerves (S1 to S5)

Coccygeal nerve

This is the body's version of networking.

Incredibly Easy miniguide to anatomy: The endocrine system

The endocrine system regulates and integrates the body's metabolic activities. This illustration shows the locations of the major endocrine glands.

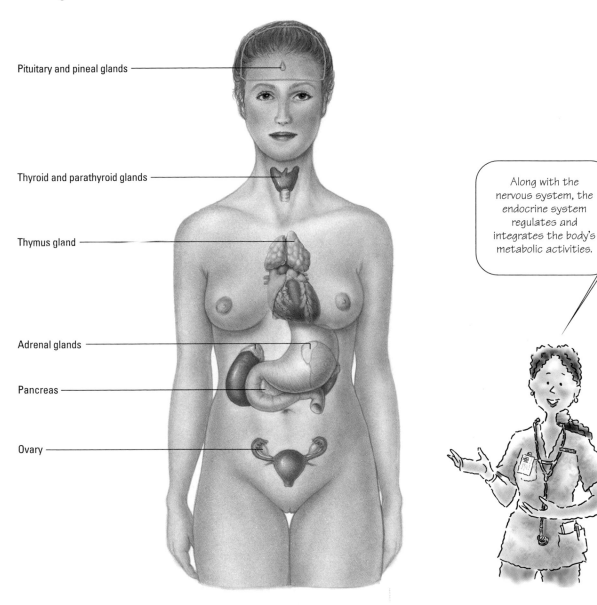

Pituitary and pineal glands

Thyroid and parathyroid glands

Thymus gland

Adrenal glands

Pancreas

Ovary

Along with the nervous system, the endocrine system regulates and integrates the body's metabolic activities.

Incredibly Easy miniguide to anatomy: The gastrointestinal system

The GI system includes the alimentary canal (pharynx, esophagus, stomach, and small and large intestines) and the accessory organs (salivary glands, liver, biliary system, and pancreas).

Esophagus

Liver

Gallbladder

Common bile duct

Stomach

Pancreas

Duodenum

Transverse colon

Ileum

Sigmoid colon

Rectum

Anus

Keep it simple. The GI tract breaks down food and fluid into simple chemicals that can be absorbed into the bloodstream and transported throughout the body.

Incredibly Easy miniguide to anatomy: The urinary system

The urinary system consists of two kidneys, two ureters, the bladder, and the urethra.

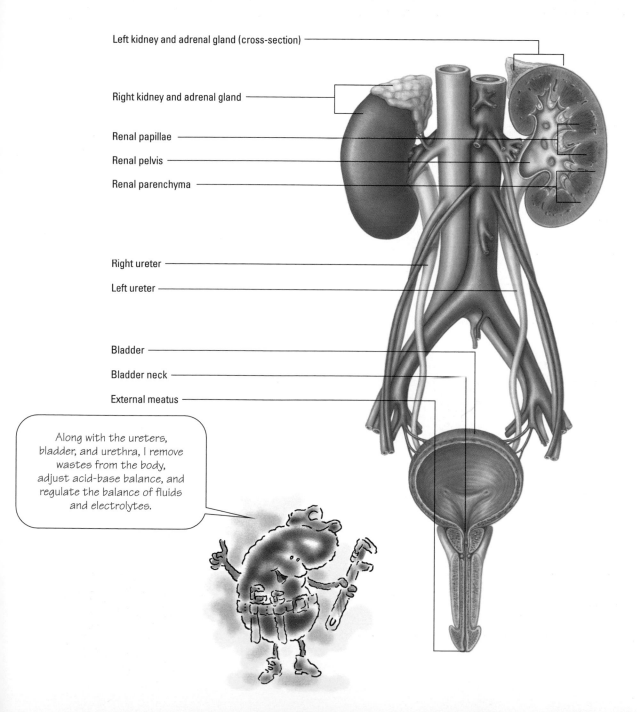

Left kidney and adrenal gland (cross-section)

Right kidney and adrenal gland

Renal papillae

Renal pelvis

Renal parenchyma

Right ureter

Left ureter

Bladder

Bladder neck

External meatus

Along with the ureters, bladder, and urethra, I remove wastes from the body, adjust acid-base balance, and regulate the balance of fluids and electrolytes.

Incredibly Easy miniguide to anatomy: The male reproductive system

The male reproductive system consists of the penis, scrotum, testes, duct system, and accessory structures (prostate gland, seminal vesicles, bulbourethral glands, and urethral glands).

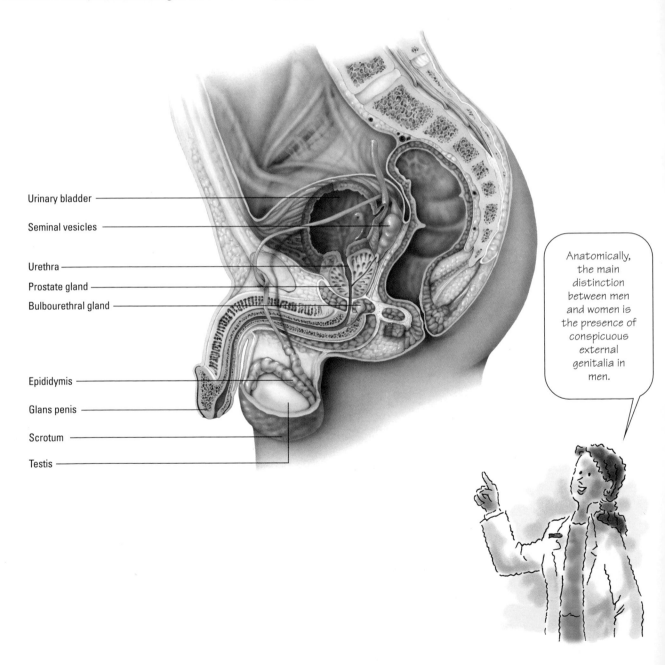

Urinary bladder

Seminal vesicles

Urethra

Prostate gland

Bulbourethral gland

Epididymis

Glans penis

Scrotum

Testis

Anatomically, the main distinction between men and women is the presence of conspicuous external genitalia in men.

Incredibly Easy miniguide to anatomy: The female reproductive system

The female reproductive system includes the vagina, uterus, fallopian tubes, ovaries, and external genitalia (not shown).

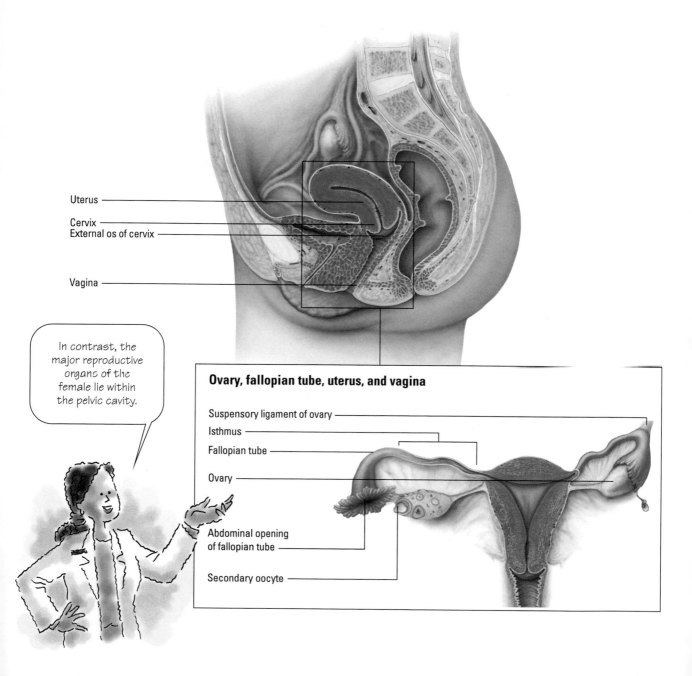

Uterus

Cervix

External os of cervix

Vagina

In contrast, the major reproductive organs of the female lie within the pelvic cavity.

Ovary, fallopian tube, uterus, and vagina

Suspensory ligament of ovary

Isthmus

Fallopian tube

Ovary

Abdominal opening of fallopian tube

Secondary oocyte

Incredibly Easy miniguide to anatomy: The skin

The skin is composed of two fused layers—the epidermis and dermis.

It's more than skin deep. The integument protects inner body structures, perceives touch, regulates body temperature, and excretes certain body fluids.

Epidermis

Dermis

Subcutaneous tissue

Stratum corneum

Granular layer (stratum granulosum)

Spinous layer (stratum spinosum)

Basal layer

Melanocyte

Sebaceous gland

Hair bulb

Eccrine sweat gland

Vertebral convergence

The two *vertebral arteries* (branches of the subclavians) converge to become the basilar artery. The *basilar artery* supplies blood to the posterior brain.

Two carotids diverged in the brain...

The common carotids branch into the two internal carotids, which divide further to supply blood to the anterior brain and the middle brain. These arteries interconnect through the *circle of Willis*, an anastomosis at the base of the brain. The circle of Willis ensures that blood continually circulates to the brain despite interruption of any of the brain's major vessels. (See *Arteries of the brain*, page 88.)

Because of the circle of Willis, blood has two paths to the brain, ensuring a continuous blood supply.

Spinal cord

The *spinal cord* is a cylindrical structure in the vertebral canal that extends from the foramen magnum at the base of the skull to the upper lumbar region of the vertebral column.

Getting on my spinal nerves

The *spinal nerves* arise from the cord. At the cord's inferior end, nerve roots cluster in the *cauda equina*.

What's the matter in the spinal cord?

Within the spinal cord, the H-shaped mass of gray matter is divided into *horns*. Horns consist mainly of neuron cell bodies. Cell bodies in the two dorsal (posterior) horns primarily relay sensations; those in the two ventral (anterior) horns play a part in voluntary and reflex motor activity. White matter surrounds the horns. This white matter consists of myelinated nerve fibers grouped in vertical columns, or *tracts*. In other words, all axons that compose one tract serve one general function, such as touch, movement, pain, and pressure. (See *A look inside the spinal cord*, page 89.)

Sensory pathways

Sensory impulses travel via the *afferent* (sensory, or ascending) *neural pathways* to the *sensory cortex* in the parietal lobe of the brain. This is where the impulses are

Zoom in

Arteries of the brain

This illustration shows the inferior surface of the brain. The anterior and posterior arteries join with smaller arteries to form the circle of Willis.

interpreted. These impulses use two major pathways: the dorsal horn and the ganglia.

Running hot and cold

Pain and temperature sensations enter the spinal cord through the *dorsal horn*. After immediately crossing over

Zoom in

A look inside the spinal cord

This cross section of the spinal cord shows an H-shaped mass of gray matter divided into horns, which consist primarily of neuron cell bodies. Cell bodies in the posterior, or dorsal, horn primarily relay information. Cell bodies in the anterior, or ventral, horn are needed for voluntary or reflex motor activity.

to the opposite side of the cord, these impulses then travel to the thalamus via the spinothalamic tract.

Feeling the pressure

Touch, pressure, and vibration sensations enter the cord via relay stations called *ganglia*. Ganglia are knotlike masses of nerve cell bodies on the dorsal roots of spinal nerves. Impulses travel up the cord in the dorsal column to the medulla, where they cross to the opposite side and enter the thalamus. The thalamus relays all incoming sensory impulses (except olfactory impulses) to the sensory cortex for interpretation.

Motor pathways

Motor impulses travel from the brain to the muscles via the *efferent* (motor, or descending) *neural pathways*.

Motor impulses originate in the *motor cortex* of the frontal lobe and reach the lower motor neurons of the peripheral nervous system via upper motor neurons.

Upper motor neurons originate in the brain and form two major systems:
- the pyramidal system
- the extrapyramidal system.

Fine tuning your response

The *pyramidal system* (corticospinal tract) is responsible for fine, skilled movements of skeletal muscle. Impulses in this system travel from the motor cortex through the internal capsule to the medulla. At the medulla, they cross to the opposite side and continue down the spinal cord.

Get your motor running

The *extrapyramidal system* (extracorticospinal tract) controls gross motor movements. Impulses originate in the premotor area of the frontal lobes and travel to the pons. At the pons, the impulses cross to the opposite side. Then the impulses travel down the spinal cord to the anterior horn, where they're relayed to the lower motor neurons. These neurons, in turn, carry the impulses to the muscles. (See *Major neural pathways*.)

Reflex responses

Reflex responses occur automatically, without any brain involvement, to protect the body. Spinal nerves, which have both sensory and motor portions, mediate *deep tendon reflexes* (involuntary contractions of a muscle after brief stretching caused by tendon percussion), *superficial reflexes* (withdrawal reflexes elicited by noxious or tactile stimulation of the skin or mucous membranes) and, in infants, *primitive reflexes*.

Deep we go

Deep tendon reflexes include reflex responses of the biceps, triceps, brachioradialis, patellar, and Achilles tendons:
- The *biceps reflex* contracts the biceps muscle and forces flexion of the forearm.
- The *triceps reflex* contracts the triceps muscle and forces extension of the forearm.

Memory jogger

To remember the difference between afferent and efferent neurons, consider this:

• Afferent neurons cause sensation to **a**scend to the brain. (Afferent neurons are sensory and ascending.)

• Efferent neurons send impulses out of the brain to **e**ffect action. (Efferent neurons are motor and descending.)

The pyramidal system is responsible for fine, skilled movements.

Now I get it!

Major neural pathways

Sensory and motor impulses travel through different pathways to the brain for interpretation.

Sensory pathways
Sensory impulses travel through two major sensory (afferent, or ascending) pathways to the sensory cortex in the cerebrum.

Motor pathways
Motor impulses travel from the motor cortex in the cerebrum to the muscles via motor (efferent, or descending) pathways.

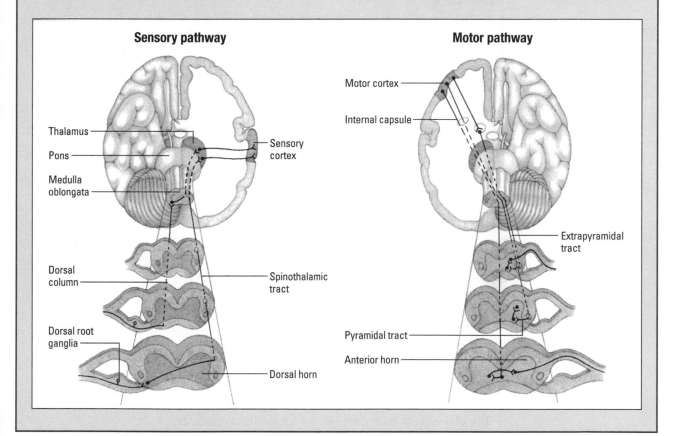

- The *brachioradialis reflex* causes supination of the hand and flexion of the forearm at the elbow.
- The *patellar reflex* forces contraction of the quadriceps muscle in the thigh with extension of the leg.

• The *Achilles reflex* forces plantar flexion of the foot at the ankle. (See *Eliciting deep tendon reflexes*.)

Rising to the superficial

Superficial reflexes are reflexes of the skin and mucous membranes. Successive attempts to stimulate these reflexes provoke increasingly limited responses. Here's a description of some superficial reflexes:

• *Plantar flexion* of the toes occurs when the lateral sole of an adult's foot is stroked from heel to great toe with a tongue blade.

• *Babinski's reflex* is an upward movement of the great toe and fanning of the little toes that occurs in children under age 2 in response to stimulation of the outer margin of the sole of the foot. This relex is an abnormal finding in adults.

• In men, the *cremasteric reflex* is stimulated by stroking the inner thigh. This forces the contraction of the cremaster muscle and elevation of the testicle on the side of the stimulus.

• The *abdominal reflexes* are induced by stroking the sides of the abdomen above and below the umbilicus, moving from the periphery toward the midline. Movement of the umbilicus toward the stimulus is normal.

Let's get primitive

Primitive reflexes are abnormal in adults but normal in infants, whose central nervous systems are immature. As the neurologic system matures, these reflexes disappear. The primitive reflexes are *grasping*, *sucking*, and *glabella*:

• The application of gentle pressure to an infant's palm results in grasping.

• An infantile sucking reflex to ingest milk is a primitive response to oral stimuli.

• The glabella reflex is elicited by repeatedly tapping the bridge of the infant's nose. The normal response is persistent blinking.

Achilles was a warrior in Homer's epic, the *Iliad*. He could only be killed by an arrow piercing the back of his heel. Therefore, the tendon located in this area is called the Achilles tendon.

Eliciting deep tendon reflexes

There are five deep tendon reflexes. Methods for eliciting these reflexes are described below.

Biceps reflex

Placing the thumb or index finger over the biceps tendon and the remaining fingers loosely over the triceps muscle, strike the thumb or index finger over the biceps tendon with the pointed end of the reflex hammer. Watch and feel for the contraction of the biceps muscle and flexion of the forearm.

Triceps reflex

Strike the triceps tendon about 2" (5 cm) above the olecranon process on the extensor surface of the upper arm. Watch for contraction of the triceps muscle and extension of the forearm.

Brachioradialis reflex

Strike the radius about 1" to 2" (2.5 to 5 cm) above the wrist and watch for supination of the hand and flexion of the forearm at the elbow.

Patellar reflex

Strike the patellar tendon just below the patella and look for contraction of the quadriceps muscle in the thigh with extension of the leg.

Achilles reflex

With the foot flexed and supporting the plantar surface, strike the Achilles tendon. Watch for plantar flexion of the foot at the ankle.

Deep tendon reflexes help protect the body.

Protective structures

The brain and spinal cord are protected from shock and infection by the bony skull and vertebrae, CSF, and three membranes: the dura mater, arachnoid membrane, and pia mater.

Dura mater

The *dura mater* is tough, fibrous, leatherlike tissue composed of two layers—the endosteal dura and meningeal dura.

The unending endosteal dura

The *endosteal dura* forms the periosteum of the skull and is continuous with the lining of the vertebral canal.

The durable meningeal dura

The *meningeal dura* is a thick membrane that covers the brain, dipping between the brain tissue and providing support and protection.

Hey, we all need a little protection sometimes!

Arachnoid membrane

The *arachnoid membrane* is a thin, fibrous membrane that hugs the brain and spinal cord, though not as precisely as the pia mater.

Pia mater

The *pia mater* is a continuous, delicate layer of connective tissue that covers and contours the spinal tissue and brain.

The spaces between

The *subdural space* lies between the dura mater and the arachnoid membrane. The *subarachnoid space* lies between the arachnoid membrane and the pia mater. Within the subarachnoid space and the brain's four ventricles is CSF, a fluid composed of water and traces of organic materials (especially protein), glucose, and electrolytes. This fluid protects the brain and spinal tissue from jolts and blows.

Peripheral nervous system

The peripheral nervous system consists of the cranial nerves, spinal nerves, and autonomic nervous system (ANS).

Cranial nerves

Twelve pairs of cranial nerves transmit motor or sensory messages (or both) primarily between the brain or brain stem and the head and neck. All cranial nerves except the olfactory and optic nerves exit from the midbrain, pons, or medulla oblongata of the brain stem. (See *Exit points for the cranial nerves*, page 96.)

Spinal nerves

Each of the 31 pairs of spinal nerves is named for the vertebra immediately below the nerve's exit point from the spinal cord. From top to bottom they're designated as C1 through S5 and the coccygeal nerve. Each spinal nerve consists of afferent (sensory) and efferent (motor) neurons, which carry messages to and from particular body regions, called *dermatomes*.

Each spinal nerve gets its name from the vertebra immediately *below* its exit point from the spinal cord.

Autonomic nervous system

The vast ANS *innervates* (supplies nerves to) all internal organs. Sometimes known as *visceral efferent nerves*, the nerves of the ANS carry messages to the viscera from the brain stem and neuroendocrine regulatory centers. The ANS has two major subdivisions: the *sympathetic* (thoracolumbar) nervous system and *parasympathetic* (craniosacral) nervous system.

When one system stimulates certain smooth muscles to contract or a gland to secrete, the other system inhibits that action. Through this dual innervation, the two divisions counterbalance each other's activities to keep body systems running smoothly.

Zoom in

Exit points for the cranial nerves

As this illustration reveals, 10 of the 12 pairs of cranial nerves (CNs) exit from the brain stem. The remaining two pairs—the olfactory and optic nerves—exit from the forebrain.

Olfactory (CN I). *Sensory:* smell

Optic (CN II). *Sensory:* vision

Trochlear (CN IV). *Motor:* extraocular eye movement (superior oblique muscles of the eyes)

Vagus (CN X). *Motor:* movement of palate, swallowing, gag reflex, activity of the thoracic and abdominal viscera, such as heart rate and peristalsis; *Sensory:* sensations of throat, larynx, and thoracic and abdominal viscera (heart, lungs, bronchi, and GI tract)

Trigeminal (CN V). *Sensory:* transmitting stimuli from face and head, corneal reflex; *Motor:* chewing, biting, and lateral jaw movements

Facial (CN VII). *Sensory:* taste receptors (anterior two-thirds of tongue); *Motor:* facial muscle movement, including muscles of expression (those in the forehead and around the eyes and mouth)

Acoustic (CN VIII). *Sensory:* hearing, sense of balance

Glossopharyngeal (CN IX). *Motor:* swallowing movements; *Sensory:* sensations of throat, taste receptors (posterior one-third of tongue)

Hypoglossal (CN XII). *Motor:* tongue movement

Spinal accessory (CN XI). *Motor:* shoulder movement, head rotation

Abducens (CN VI). *Motor:* extraocular eye movement (lateral)

Oculomotor (CN III). *Motor:* extraocular eye movement (superior, medial, and inferior lateral), pupillary constriction, upper eyelid elevation

Sympathetic nervous system

Sympathetic nerves called *preganglionic neurons* exit the spinal cord between the levels of the first thoracic and second lumbar vertebrae.

Ganglia branch out

When they leave the spinal cord, preganglionic neurons enter small ganglia near the cord. The ganglia form a chain that spreads the impulse to *postganglionic neurons.* Postganglionic neurons reach many organs and glands and can produce widespread, generalized physiologic responses. These responses include:
• vasoconstriction
• elevated blood pressure
• enhanced blood flow to skeletal muscles
• increased heart rate and contractility
• increased respiratory rate
• smooth-muscle relaxation of the bronchioles, GI tract, and urinary tract
• sphincter contraction
• pupillary dilation and ciliary muscle relaxation
• increased sweat gland secretion
• reduced pancreatic secretion.

My postganglionic neurons are making my blood pressure rise!

Parasympathetic nervous system

Fibers of the parasympathetic nervous system leave the CNS by way of the cranial nerves from the midbrain and

Faster! Get with the program!

The sympathetic and parasympathetic nervous systems work together by sending complementary signals.

You can take it easy now.

medulla and the spinal nerves between the second and fourth sacral vertebrae (S2 to S4).

See ya later, CNS

After leaving the CNS, the long preganglionic fiber of each parasympathetic nerve travels to a ganglion near a particular organ or gland. The short postganglionic fiber enters the organ or gland. This creates a more specific response involving only one organ or gland.

Such a response might be:
• reduction in heart rate, contractility, and conduction velocity
• bronchial smooth-muscle constriction
• increased GI tract tone and peristalsis, with sphincter relaxation
• increased bladder tone and urinary system sphincter relaxation
• vasodilation of external genitalia, causing erection
• pupil constriction
• increased pancreatic, salivary, and lacrimal secretions.

Special sense organs

Sensory stimulation allows the body to interact with the environment. The distal ends of the dendrites of sensory neurons serve as sensory receptors, sending messages to the brain. The brain also receives stimulation from the special sense organs—the eyes, ears, and gustatory and olfactory organs.

Eye

The *eye* is the organ of vision. It contains about 70% of the body's sensory receptors. Although the eye measures about 1″ (2.5 cm) in diameter, only its anterior surface is visible.

Extraocular eye structure

Extraocular muscles hold the eyes in place and control their movement. Their coordinated action keeps both eyes parallel and creates binocular vision. These muscles have mutually antagonistic actions: As one muscle contracts, its opposing muscle relaxes.

Extraocular structures include the eyelids, conjunctivae, and lacrimal apparatus. Together with the extraocular muscles, these structures support and protect the eyeball.

Eyelids

The *eyelids* (also called the *palpebrae*) are loose folds of skin that cover the anterior portion of the eye. The lid margins contain hair follicles, which contain eyelashes and sebaceous glands.

In the blink of an eye

When open, the upper eyelid extends beyond the *limbus* (the junction of the cornea and the sclera) and covers a small portion of the iris.

The eyelids contain three types of glands:
• *meibomian glands* — sebaceous glands that secrete sebum, an oily substance that keeps the eye lubricated
• *glands of Zeis* — modified sebaceous glands connected to the follicles of the eyelashes
• *Moll's glands* — ordinary sweat glands.

When closed, the upper and lower eyelids cover the eye completely.

Conjunctivae

Conjunctivae are thin mucous membranes that line the inner surface of each eyelid and the anterior portion of the sclera. Conjunctivae guard the eye from invasion by foreign matter. The *palpebral conjunctiva* — the portion that lines the inner surface of the eyelids — appears shiny pink or red. The *bulbar* (or ocular) *conjunctiva*, which joins the palpebral portion and covers the exposed part of the sclera, contains many small, normally visible blood vessels.

Lacrimal apparatus

The structures of the *lacrimal apparatus* (lacrimal glands, punctum, lacrimal sac, and nasolacrimal duct) lubricate and protect the cornea and conjunctivae by producing and absorbing tears. Tears keep the cornea and conjunctivae moist. Tears also contain *lysozyme*, an enzyme that protects against bacterial invasion.

The eyelid protects the eye, regulates the entrance of light, and distributes tears over the eye.

Zoom in

A close look at tears

Tears begin in the lacrimal gland and drain through the nasolacrimal duct into the nose.

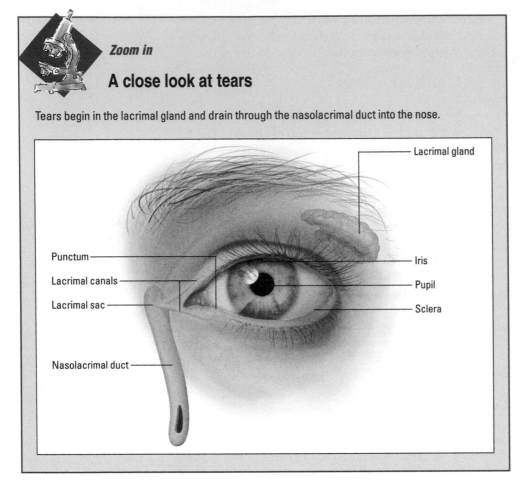

Lacrimal gland

Punctum

Lacrimal canals

Lacrimal sac

Iris

Pupil

Sclera

Nasolacrimal duct

These darn tears will be the death of me!

Cry me a river

As the eyelids blink, they direct the flow of tears from the lacrimal ducts to the *inner canthus*, the medial angle between the eyelids. Tears pool at the inner canthus and drain through the *punctum*, a tiny opening. From there they flow through the *lacrimal canals* into the lacrimal sac. Lastly, they drain through the nasolacrimal duct and into the nose. (See *A close look at tears*.)

Intraocular eye structures

Intraocular structures within the eyeball are directly involved with vision. (See *Looking at intraocular structures*.)

Zoom in

Looking at intraocular structures

Some intraocular structures, such as the sclera, cornea, iris, pupil, and anterior chamber, are visible to the naked eye. Others, such as the retina, are visible only with an ophthalmoscope. These illustrations show the major structures within the eye.

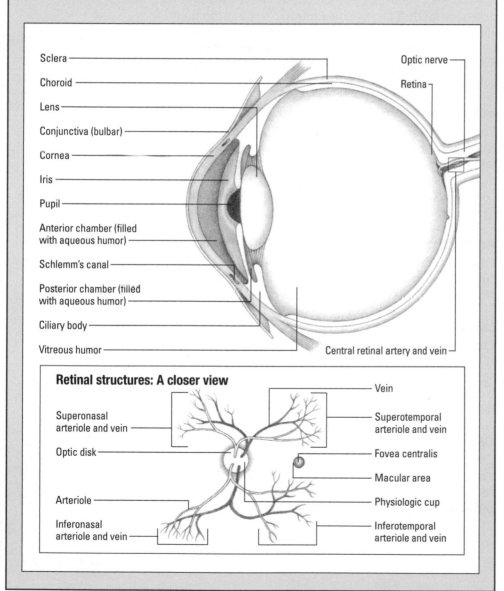

Sclera

Choroid

Lens

Conjunctiva (bulbar)

Cornea

Iris

Pupil

Anterior chamber (filled with aqueous humor)

Schlemm's canal

Posterior chamber (filled with aqueous humor)

Ciliary body

Vitreous humor

Optic nerve

Retina

Central retinal artery and vein

Retinal structures: A closer view

Superonasal arteriole and vein

Optic disk

Arteriole

Inferonasal arteriole and vein

Vein

Superotemporal arteriole and vein

Fovea centralis

Macular area

Physiologic cup

Inferotemporal arteriole and vein

Want to see the sclera, cornea, iris, or pupil? Just look in the mirror.

The sclera, cornea, iris, pupil, anterior chamber, aqueous humor, lens, ciliary body, and posterior chamber are found in the anterior segment. The vitreous humor, posterior sclera, choroid, and retina are found in the posterior segment.

Sclera and cornea

The white *sclera* coats four-fifths of the outside of the eyeball, maintaining its size and form. The *cornea* is continuous with the sclera at the limbus, revealing the pupil and iris. A smooth, transparent tissue, the cornea has no blood supply. The corneal epithelium merges with the bulbar conjunctiva at the limbus. The cornea is highly sensitive to touch and is kept moist by tears.

Iris and pupil

The *iris* is a circular contractile disk that contains smooth and radial muscles. It has an opening in the center for the *pupil*. Eye color depends on the amount of pigment in the endothelial layers of the iris. Pupil size is controlled by involuntary dilatory and sphincter muscles in the posterior region of the iris that regulate light entry.

Anterior chamber and aqueous humor

The *anterior chamber* is a cavity bounded in front by the cornea and behind by the lens and iris. It's filled with a clear, watery fluid called *aqueous humor*.

Lens

The *lens* is situated directly behind the iris at the pupillary opening. Composed of transparent fibers in an elastic membrane called the *lens capsule*, the lens acts like a camera lens, refracting and focusing light onto the retina.

Ciliary body

The *ciliary body* (three muscles along with the iris that make up the anterior part of the vascular uveal tract) controls the lens thickness. Together with the coordinated action of muscles

Moisture plays an important role in the eye. For example, tears protect the cornea by keeping it moist.

in the iris, the ciliary body regulates the light focused through the lens onto the retina.

Posterior chamber

The *posterior chamber* is a small space directly posterior to the iris but anterior to the lens. It's filled with aqueous humor.

Vitreous humor

The *vitreous humor* consists of a thick, gelatinous material that fills the space behind the lens. There, it maintains placement of the retina and the spherical shape of the eyeball.

Posterior sclera and choroid

The *posterior sclera* is a white, opaque, fibrous layer that covers the posterior segment of the eyeball. It continues back to the dural sheath, covering the optic nerve. The *choroid* lies beneath the posterior sclera. It contains many small arteries and veins.

Retina

The *retina* is the innermost coat of the eyeball. It receives visual stimuli and sends them to the brain. Each of the four sets of retinal vessels contains a transparent arteriole and vein as well as the optic disk, the physiologic cup, rods and cones, and the macula.

The posterior segment of the eye has three layers: fibrous, vascular, and sensory.

The optimal optic disk

Arterioles and veins become progressively thinner as they leave the optic disk. The *optic disk* is a well-defined, 1.5-mm round or oval area on the retina. Creamy yellow to pink in color, the optic disk allows the optic nerve to enter the retina at a point called the *nerve head*. A whitish to grayish crescent of scleral tissue may be present on the lateral side of the disk.

The cup within the disk

The *physiologic cup* is a light-colored depression within the optic disk on the temporal side. It covers one-third of the center of the disk.

Visionaries

Photoreceptor neurons called *rods* and *cones* compose the visual receptors of the retina. These receptors are responsible for vision.

Count macula

The *macula* is lateral to the optic disk. It's slightly darker than the rest of the retina and without visible retinal vessels. A slight depression in the center of the macula, known as the *fovea centralis*, contains the heaviest concentration of cones and is a main receptor for vision and color.

Vision pathway

Intraocular structures perceive and form images and then send them to the brain for interpretation. To interpret these images properly, the brain relies on structures along the vision pathway. The *vision pathway* uses the optic nerve, optic chiasm, and retina to create the proper visual fields.

The optic disk has no light receptors and is therefore a "blind spot." But I compensate so that there's usually no apparent gap in what is seen.

Criss-crossing tracts

In the *optic chiasm*, fibers from the nasal aspects of both retinas cross to the opposite sides, and fibers from the temporal portions remain uncrossed. These crossed and uncrossed fibers form the *optic tracts*. Injury to one of the optic nerves can cause blindness in the corresponding eye. An injury or lesion in the optic chiasm can cause partial vision loss (for example, loss of the two temporal visual fields).

Focusing on the fovea centralis

Image formation begins when eye structures refract light rays from an object. Normally, the cornea, aqueous humor, lens, and vitreous humor refract light rays from an object, focusing them on the fovea centralis, where an inverted and reversed image clearly forms. Within the retina, rods and cones turn the projected image into an impulse and transmit it to the optic nerve.

I see! We turn projected images into impulses that we then transmit to the optic nerve.

Follow the tracts to the cerebral cortex

The impulse travels to the optic chiasm, (where the two optic nerves unite and split again into two optic tracts) and then continues into the optic section of the cerebral cortex. There, the inverted and reversed image on the retina is processed by the brain to create an image as it truly appears in the field of vision.

Ear

The *ears* are the organs of hearing. They also maintain the body's equilibrium. The ear is divided into three main parts: external, middle, and inner. (See *Ear structures*, page 106.)

External ear structures

The *external ear* consists of the *auricle* (pinna) and the *external auditory canal*. The *mastoid process* isn't part of the external ear but is an important bony landmark behind the lower part of the auricle.

Middle ear structures

The *middle ear* is also called the *tympanic cavity*. It's an air-filled cavity within the hard portion of the temporal bone. The tympanic cavity is lined with mucosa. It's bound distally by the tympanic membrane and medially by the oval and round windows.

Tympanic membrane

The *tympanic membrane* consists of layers of skin, fibrous tissue, and a mucous membrane. It transmits sound vibrations to the internal ear.

Eustachian tube

The *eustachian*, or auditory, *tube* extends downward, forward, and inward from the middle ear cavity to the nasopharynx. It has a useful function: It allows the pressure against inner and outer surfaces of the tympanic membrane to equalize, preventing rupture.

Oval window

The *oval window* (fenestra ovalis) is an opening in the wall between the middle and inner ears into which part of the *stapes* (a tiny bone of the middle ear) fits. It transmits vibrations to the inner ear.

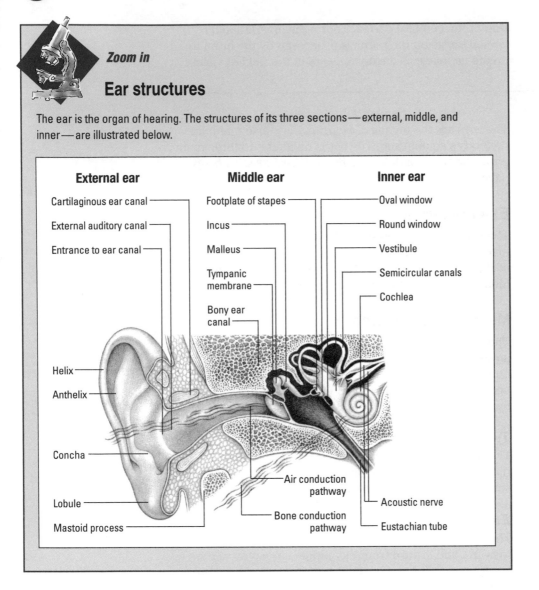

Zoom in

Ear structures

The ear is the organ of hearing. The structures of its three sections—external, middle, and inner—are illustrated below.

External ear
- Cartilaginous ear canal
- External auditory canal
- Entrance to ear canal
- Helix
- Anthelix
- Concha
- Lobule
- Mastoid process

Middle ear
- Footplate of stapes
- Incus
- Malleus
- Tympanic membrane
- Bony ear canal
- Air conduction pathway
- Bone conduction pathway

Inner ear
- Oval window
- Round window
- Vestibule
- Semicircular canals
- Cochlea
- Acoustic nerve
- Eustachian tube

Round window

The *round window* (fenestra cochleae) is another opening in the same wall. It's enclosed by the secondary tympanic membrane. Like the oval window, the round window transmits vibrations to the inner ear.

Small bones

The middle ear contains three small bones, called *ossicles*, that conduct vibratory motion of the tympanum to the oval window. The ossicles are:

- the *malleus* (hammer), which attaches to the tympanic membrane and transfers sound to the incus
- the *incus* (anvil), which articulates the malleus and the stapes and carries vibration to the stapes
- the *stapes* (stirrup), which connects vibratory motion from the incus to the oval window.

Inner ear structures

In the inner ear, vibration excites receptor nerve endings. A bony labyrinth and a membranous labyrinth combine to form the inner ear. The inner ear contains the vestibule, cochlea, and semicircular canals.

Vestibule

The *vestibule* is located posterior to the cochlea and anterior to the semicircular canals. It serves as the entrance to the inner ear. It houses two membranous sacs, the *saccule* and *utricle*. Suspended in a fluid called *perilymph*, the saccule and utricle sense gravity changes and linear and angular acceleration.

Cochlea

The *cochlea*, a bony, spiraling cone, extends from the anterior part of the vestibule. Within it lies the *cochlear duct*, a triangular, membranous structure that houses the *organ of Corti*. The receptor organ for hearing, the organ of Corti transmits sound to the cochlear branch of the acoustic nerve (CN VIII).

Semicircular canals

The three *semicircular canals* project from the posterior aspect of the vestibule. Each canal is oriented in one of three planes: superior, posterior, and lateral. The *semicircular duct* traverses the canals and connects with the utricle anteriorly. The *crista ampullaris* sits at the end of each canal and contains hair cells and support cells. It's stimulated by sudden movements or changes in the rate or direction of movement.

Hearing pathways

For hearing to occur, sound waves travel through the ear by two pathways—air conduction and bone conduction:

• *Air conduction* occurs when sound waves travel in the air through the external and middle ear to the inner ear.
• *Bone conduction* occurs when sound waves travel through bone to the inner ear.

For hearing to occur, sound waves travel through the ear by two pathways — air conduction and bone conduction.

Interpreting the vibrations, man

Vibrations transmitted through air and bone stimulate nerve impulses in the inner ear. The cochlear branch of the acoustic nerve transmits these vibrations to the auditory area of the cerebral cortex. The cerebral cortex then interprets the sound.

Nose and mouth

The *nose* is the sense organ for smell. The mucosal epithelium that lines the uppermost portion of the nasal cavity houses receptors for fibers of the olfactory nerve (CN I).

Good old olfactory

These receptors, called *olfactory* (smell) *receptors*, consist of hair cells, which are highly sensitive but easily fatigued. They're stimulated by the slightest odors but stop sensing even the strongest smells after a short time.

Slip of the tongue

The tongue and the roof of the mouth contain most of the receptors for the taste nerve fibers (located in branches of CNs VII and IX). Called *taste buds*, these receptors are stimulated by chemicals. They respond to four taste sensations: sweet, sour, bitter, and salty. All the other flavors a person senses result from a combination of olfactory-receptor and taste-bud stimulation.

Quick quiz

1. The components of the central nervous system include:
  A. the spinal cord and cranial nerves.
  B. the brain and spinal cord.
  C. the sympathetic and parasympathetic nervous systems.
  D. the cranial nerves and spinal nerves.

Answer: B. The two main divisions of the nervous system are the CNS, which includes the brain and spinal cord, and the peripheral nervous system, which consists of the cranial nerves, spinal nerves, and ANS.

2. The brain is protected from shock and infection by:
  A. bones, the meninges, and CSF.
  B. gray matter, bones, and the primitive structures.
  C. the blood-brain barrier, CSF, and white matter.
  D. axons, neurons, and meninges.

Answer: A. Bones (the skull and vertebral column), the meninges, and CSF protect the brain from shock and infection.

3. The visual receptors of the retina are composed of:
  A. the pupil and lens.
  B. the optic disk and optic nerve.
  C. vitreous humor and aqueous humor.
  D. rods and cones.

Answer: D. Photoreceptor neurons called rods and cones compose the visual receptors of the retina.

4. The external ear consists of:
  A. the vestibule, cochlea, and semicircular ducts.
  B. the tympanic membrane, oval window, and round window.
  C. the auricle and external auditory canal.
  D. the malleus, incus, and stapes.

Answer: C. The auricle and external auditory canal are part of the external ear.

5. The cranial nerves transmit motor and sensory messages between the:
- A. spine and body dermatomes.
- B. brain and the head and neck.
- C. viscera and the brain.
- D. brain and skeletal muscles.

Answer: B. The 12 pairs of cranial nerves transmit motor (efferent) and sensory (afferent) messages between the brain or brain stem and the head and neck.

Scoring

☆☆☆   If you answered all five questions correctly, stupendous! You're definitely brainy.

☆☆   If you answered four questions correctly, remarkable. Your gray matter is working at lightning speed.

☆   If you answered fewer than four questions correctly, don't get nervous. Give your brain another workout by reviewing the chapter again.

Endocrine system

Just the facts

In this chapter, you'll learn:

♦ the functions of endocrine glands

♦ hormone release and transportation in the endocrine system

♦ the role of receptors in the influence of hormones on cells.

A look at the endocrine system

The three major components of the endocrine system are:
• *glands* — specialized cell clusters or organs
• *hormones* — chemical substances secreted by glands in response to stimulation
• *receptors* — protein molecules that bind specifically with other molecules, such as hormones, to trigger specific physiologic changes in a target cell.

Glands

The major glands of the endocrine system are:
• pituitary gland
• thyroid gland
• parathyroid glands
• adrenal glands
• pancreas
• thymus
• pineal gland
• gonads (ovaries and testes). (See *Components of the endocrine system*, page 112.)

Along with the nervous system, the endocrine system regulates and integrates the body's metabolic activities.

Body shop

Components of the endocrine system

Endocrine glands secrete hormones directly into the bloodstream to regulate body function. This illustration shows the location of the major endocrine glands (except the gonads).

- Pineal gland
- Pituitary gland
- Thyroid gland
- Thymus
- Adrenal glands
- Pancreas

The pituitary gland

The *pituitary gland* (also called the *hypophysis* or *master gland*) rests in the *sella turcica*, a depression in the sphenoid bone at the base of the brain. This pea-sized gland connects with the hypothalamus via the infundibulum, from which it receives chemical and nervous stimu-

Now I get it!

How the hypothalamus affects endocrine activities

The *hypothalamus* is the integrative center for the endocrine and autonomic (involuntary) nervous systems. It helps control some endocrine glands by neural and hormonal stimulation.

Take the path

Neural pathways connect the hypothalamus to the posterior pituitary gland. These hypothalamic neurons stimulate the posterior pituitary gland to secrete two effector hormones—antidiuretic hormone (ADH) and oxytocin—which are stored in the posterior pituitary.

What happens after secretion

When ADH is secreted, the body retains water. Oxytocin stimulates uterine contractions during labor and milk secretion in lactating women.

The regulator

The hypothalamus also produces many other inhibiting and stimulating hormones and other factors, which it uses to regulate functions of the anterior pituitary.

> The hypothalamus is the integrative center for the endocrine and autonomic nervous systems.

lation. (See *How the hypothalamus affects endocrine activities.*)

Anterior pituitary

The pituitary has two main regions. The *anterior pituitary* (adenohypophysis) is the larger region. It produces at least six hormones:
- growth hormone (GH), or somatotropin
- thyroid-stimulating hormone (TSH), or thyrotropin
- corticotropin
- follicle-stimulating hormone (FSH)
- luteinizing hormone (LH)
- prolactin.

Posterior pituitary

The *posterior pituitary* makes up about 25% of the gland. It serves as a storage area for antidiuretic hormone (ADH), also known as *vasopressin,* and oxytocin, which are produced by the hypothalamus.

Thyroid gland

The *thyroid* lies directly below the larynx, partially in front of the trachea. Its two lateral lobes—one on either side of the trachea—join with a narrow tissue bridge, called the *isthmus*, to give the gland its butterfly shape.

Two lobes that function as one

The two lobes of the thyroid function as one unit to produce the hormones *triiodothyronine (T_3)*, *thyroxine (T_4)*, and *calcitonin*.

T_3 and T_4 equal thyroid hormone

T_3 and T_4 are collectively referred to as *thyroid hormone*. The body's major metabolic hormone, thyroid hormone, regulates metabolism by speeding cellular respiration.

Calcium balancing act

Calcitonin maintains the calcium level of blood. It does this by inhibiting the release of calcium from bone. Secretion of calcitonin is controlled by the calcium concentration of the fluid surrounding the thyroid cells.

Parathyroid glands

The *parathyroid glands* are the body's smallest known endocrine glands. These glands are embedded on the posterior surface of the thyroid, one in each corner.

Calcium cohort

Working together as a single gland, the parathyroid glands produce *parathyroid hormone* (PTH). The main function of PTH is to help regulate the blood's calcium balance. This hormone adjusts the rate at which calcium and magnesium ions are lost in the urine. PTH also increases the movement of phosphate ions from the blood to urine for excretion.

Adrenal glands

The two *adrenal glands* each lie on top of a kidney. These almond-shaped glands contain two distinct structures — the adrenal cortex and the adrenal medulla — that function as separate endocrine glands.

Adrenal cortex

The *adrenal cortex* is the large outer layer. It forms the bulk of the adrenal gland. It has three zones, or cell layers:

The *zona glomerulosa*, the outermost zone, produces mineralocorticoids (primarily aldosterone) that help maintain fluid balance by increasing sodium reabsorption.

The *zona fasciculata*, the middle and largest zone, produces the glucocorticoids cortisol (hydrocortisone), cortisone, and corticosterone as well as small amounts of the sex hormones androgen and estrogen. Glucocorticoids help regulate metabolism and resistance to stress.

The *zona reticularis*, the innermost zone, produces some sex hormones.

It's fascinating, really. The zona fasciculata produces cortisol, cortisone, corticosterone, and even small amounts of androgen and estrogen.

Adrenal medulla

The *adrenal medulla*, or inner layer of the adrenal gland, functions as part of the sympathetic nervous system and produces two catecholamines: epinephrine and norepinephrine. Because catecholamines play an important role in the autonomic nervous system (ANS), the adrenal medulla is considered a neuroendocrine structure.

Pancreas

The *pancreas*, a triangular organ, is nestled in the curve of the duodenum, stretching horizontally behind the stomach and extending to the spleen.

Endo and exo

The pancreas performs both endocrine and exocrine functions. *Acinar cells* make up most of the gland and regulate pancreatic exocrine function.

Islands in an acinar sea

The endocrine cells of the pancreas are called the *islet cells*, or *islets of Langerhans*. These cells exist in clusters and are found scattered among the acinar cells. The islets contain alpha, beta, and delta cells that produce important hormones:

• Alpha cells produce *glucagon*, a hormone that raises the blood glucose level by triggering the breakdown of glycogen to glucose.

• Beta cells produce *insulin*. Insulin lowers the blood glucose level by stimulating the conversion of glucose to glycogen.

• Delta cells produce *somatostatin*. Somatostatin inhibits the release of GH, corticotropin, and certain other hormones.

I'm an alpha cell, the glucagon producer.

I'm a beta cell, an insulin producer.

I guess I'm a delta cell, the somatostatin producer.

Thymus

The *thymus* is located below the sternum and contains lymphatic tissue. It reaches maximal size at puberty and then starts to atrophy.

Producing Mr. T cells, fool!

Because the thymus produces T cells, which are important in cell-mediated immunity, its major role seems to be related to the immune system. However, the thymus also produces the peptide hormones thymosin and thymopoietin. These hormones promote growth of peripheral lymphoid tissue.

That's really neat. I didn't know I was made in the thymus.

Pineal gland

The tiny *pineal gland* lies at the back of the third ventricle of the brain. It produces the hormone *melatonin*, primarily during the dark hours of the day. Little hormone is produced during daytime hours, thereby influencing sleep-wake cycles. Melatonin is thought to regulate cicadian rhythms, body temperature, cardiovascular function, and reproduction.

Gonads

The *gonads* include the ovaries (in females) and the testes (in males).

Ovaries

The *ovaries* are paired, oval glands that are situated on either side of the uterus. They produce ova (eggs) and the steroidal hormones estrogen and progesterone. These hormones have four functions:

They promote development and maintenance of female sex characteristics.

They regulate the menstrual cycle.

They maintain the uterus for pregnancy.

Along with other hormones, they prepare the mammary glands for lactation.

Testes

The *testes* are paired structures that lie in an extra-abdominal pouch (scrotum) in the male. They produce spermatozoa and the male sex hormone testosterone. Testosterone stimulates and maintains masculine sex characteristics and triggers the male sex drive.

Hormones

Hormones are complex chemical substances that trigger or regulate the activity of an organ or a group of cells. Hormones are classified by their molecular structure as polypeptides, steroids, or amines.

Polypeptides

Polypeptides are protein compounds made of many amino acids that are connected by peptide bonds. They include:
• anterior pituitary hormones (GH, TSH, corticotropin, FSH, LH, and prolactin)
• posterior pituitary hormones (ADH and oxytocin)
• parathyroid hormone (PTH)
• pancreatic hormones (insulin and glucagon).

Steroids

Steroids are derived from cholesterol. They include:
• adrenocortical hormones secreted by the adrenal cortex (aldosterone and cortisol)
• sex hormones secreted by the gonads (estrogen and progesterone in females and testosterone in males).

Amines

Amines are derived from *tyrosine*, an essential amino acid found in most proteins. They include:
• thyroid hormones (T_4 and T_3)
• catecholamines (epinephrine, norepinephrine, and dopamine).

Hormone release and transport

Although all hormone release results from endocrine gland stimulation, release patterns of hormones vary greatly. For example:
• corticotropin (secreted by the anterior pituitary) and cortisol (secreted by the adrenal cortex) are released in

spurts in response to body rhythm cycles. Levels of these hormones peak in the morning.
• Secretion of PTH (by the parathyroid gland) and prolactin (by the anterior pituitary) occurs fairly evenly throughout the day.
• Secretion of insulin by the pancreas can occur at a steady rate or sporadically, depending on blood glucose levels.

Thyroid and steroid hormones circulate while bound to plasma proteins, whereas catecholamines and most polypeptides aren't protein-bound.

Hormonal action

When a hormone reaches its target site, it binds to a specific receptor on the cell membrane or within the cell. Polypeptides and some amines bind to membrane receptor sites. The smaller, more lipid-soluble steroids and thyroid hormones diffuse through the cell membrane and bind to intracellular receptors.

Right on target!

After binding occurs, each hormone produces unique physiologic changes, depending on its target site and its specific action at that site. A particular hormone may have different effects at different target sites.

Hormonal regulation

To maintain the body's delicate equilibrium, a feedback mechanism regulates hormone production and secretion. The mechanism involves hormones, blood chemicals and metabolites, and the nervous system. This system may be simple or complex. (See *The feedback loop*, page 120.)

Signaling secretory cells

For normal function, each gland must contain enough appropriately programmed secretory cells to release active hormones on demand. Secretory cells need supervision. A secretory cell can't sense on its own when to release the hormone or how much to release. It gets this information from sensing and signaling systems that integrate many messages. Together, stimulatory and inhibitory signals actively control the rate and duration of hormone release.

When released, the hormone travels to *target cells*, where a receptor molecule recognizes it and binds to it. (See *A close look at target cells*, page 121.)

Now I get it!

The feedback loop

This diagram shows the negative feedback mechanism that helps regulate the endocrine system.

From simple...

Simple feedback occurs when the level of one substance regulates the secretion of hormones (simple loop). For example, a low serum calcium level stimulates the parathyroid gland to release parathyroid hormone (PTH). PTH, in turn, promotes resorption of calcium from the GI tract, kidneys, and bones. A high serum calcium level inhibits PTH secretion.

...to complex

When the hypothalamus receives negative feedback from target glands, the mechanism is more complicated (complex loop). *Complex feedback* occurs through an axis established between the hypothalamus, pituitary gland, and target organ. For example, secretion of corticotropin-releasing hormone from the hypothalamus stimulates release of corticotropin by the pituitary gland, which in turn stimulates cortisol secretion by the adrenal gland (the target organ). A rise in serum cortisol levels inhibits corticotropin secretion by decreasing corticotropin-releasing hormone.

Feedback refers to information sent to endocrine glands, signaling the need for changes in hormone levels.

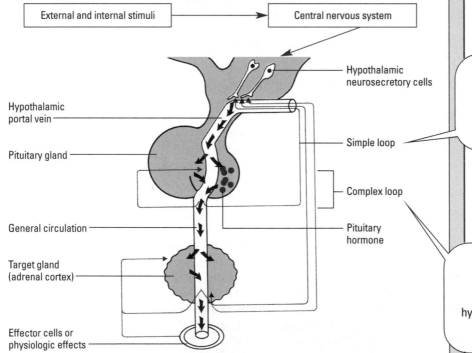

Simple feedback occurs when the level of one substance regulates the secretion of hormones.

Complex feedback occurs through an axis established between the hypothalamus, pituitary gland, and target organ.

Now I get it!

A close look at target cells

A hormone acts only on cells that have receptors specific to that hormone. The sensitivity of a target cell depends on how many receptors it has for a particular hormone. The more receptor sites, the more sensitive the target cell.

Capillary

Circulating blood

Hormone

Target cells

Nontarget cells

Extracellular and intracellular receptors

A hormone acts only on a cell that has a receptor specific to that hormone.

Mechanisms that control hormone release

Four basic mechanisms control hormone release:

- the pituitary–target gland axis
- the hypothalamic-pituitary–target gland axis
- chemical regulation
- nervous system regulation.

Pituitary-target gland axis

The pituitary gland regulates other endocrine glands —
and their hormones — through secretion of *trophic hormones* (releasing and inhibiting hormones). These
hormones include:
• corticotropin, which regulates adrenocortical hormones
• TSH, which regulates T_4 and T_3
• LH, which regulates gonadal hormones.

Picking up feedback

The pituitary gland gets feedback about target glands by
continuously monitoring levels of hormones produced by
these glands. If a change occurs, the pituitary gland corrects it in one of two ways:
• by increasing the trophic hormones, which stimulate
the target gland to increase production of target gland
hormones
• by decreasing the trophic hormones, thereby decreasing target gland stimulation and target gland hormone
levels.

Hypothalamic-pituitary-target gland axis

The hypothalamus also produces trophic hormones that
regulate anterior pituitary hormones. By controlling anterior pituitary hormones, which regulate the target gland
hormones, the hypothalamus affects target glands as well.

Chemical regulation

Endocrine glands not controlled by the pituitary gland
may be controlled by specific substances that trigger
gland secretions. For example, blood glucose level is a
major regulator of glucagon and insulin release. When
blood glucose level rises, the pancreas is stimulated to in-crease insulin secretion and suppress glucagon secretion.
A depressed level of blood glucose, on the other hand,
triggers increased glucagon secretion and suppresses insulin secretion. (See *Endocrine changes with aging.*)

Nervous system regulation

The central nervous system (CNS) helps to regulate hormone secretion in several ways.

Specific
substances,
such as blood
glucose, can
trigger gland
secretions.

Hypothalamus has control...

The hypothalamus controls pituitary hormones. Because hypothalamic nerve cells stimulate the posterior pituitary to secrete ADH and oxytocin, these hormones are controlled directly by the CNS.

...but stimuli matter, too

Nervous system stimuli—such as hypoxia (oxygen deficiency), nausea, pain, stress, and certain drugs—also affect ADH levels.

ANS steers this ship...

The ANS controls catecholamine secretion by the adrenal medulla.

...while stress spikes corticotropin

The nervous system also affects other endocrine hormones. For example, stress, which leads to sympathetic stimulation, causes the pituitary to release corticotropin.

Quick quiz

1. The purpose of the endocrine system is to:
   A. deliver nutrients to the body's cells.
   B. regulate and integrate the body's metabolic activities.
   C. eliminate waste products from the body.
   D. control the body's temperature and produce blood cells.

Answer: B. Along with the nervous system, the endocrine system regulates and integrates the body's metabolic activities.

2. The mechanism that helps regulate the endocrine system is called the:
   A. transport mechanism.
   B. self-regulation mechanism.
   C. feedback mechanism.
   D. pituitary-target gland axis.

Answer: C. The negative feedback mechanism helps regulate the endocrine system by signaling to the endocrine glands the need for changes in hormone levels.

Senior moment

Endocrine changes with aging

As a person ages, normal changes in endocrine function include reduced progesterone production, a 50% decline in serum aldosterone levels, and a 25% decrease in cortisol secretion rate.

Another common and important endocrine change in elderly people is a change in glucose metabolism in response to stress. Normally, both young adults and the elderly have similar fasting blood glucose levels. However, under stressful conditions, an elderly person's blood glucose level rises higher and remains elevated longer than does a younger adult's.

3. The gland that produces glucagon is the:
   A.   pancreas.
   B.   thymus.
   C.   adrenal gland.
   D.   pituitary gland.

Answer: A. The alpha cells of the pancreas produce glucagon, a hormone that raises the blood glucose level by triggering the breakdown of glycogen to glucose.

4. Pituitary hormones are controlled by the:
   A.   pancreas.
   B.   hypothalamus.
   C.   thyroid gland.
   D.   parathyroid glands.

Answer: B. The hypothalamus controls pituitary hormones.

Scoring

☆☆☆   If you answered all four questions correctly, astonishing! Your brain cells must be on steroids!

☆☆   If you answered three questions correctly, bon voyage! You've just won a trip to the islets of Langerhans!

☆   If you answered fewer than three questions correctly, don't moan over these hormones. Focus your energy on the chapter ahead.

8

Cardiovascular system

Just the facts

In this chapter, you'll learn:

♦ structures of the heart and their functions

♦ the heart's conduction system

♦ the flow of blood through the heart and the body.

A look at the cardiovascular system

The cardiovascular system (sometimes called the *circulatory system*) consists of the *heart, blood vessels,* and *lymphatics.* This network brings life-sustaining oxygen and nutrients to the body's cells, removes metabolic waste products, and carries hormones from one part of the body to another.

Doing double duty

The heart is actually two separate pumps: The right side pumps the blood to the lungs, and the left side pumps the blood to the rest of the body.

Where the heart lies

About the size of a closed fist, the heart lies beneath the sternum in the *mediastinum* (the cavity between the lungs), between the second and sixth ribs. In most people, the heart rests obliquely, with its right side below and almost in front of the left. Because of its oblique angle, the heart's broad part or top is at its upper right, and its pointed end (apex) is at its

> The angle at which I lie in the chest varies according to body build. In a tall, thin person, I'm more vertical than in a short, stocky person.

lower left. The apex is the *point of maximal impulse*, where the heart sounds are the loudest.

Heart structure

Surrounded by a sac called the *pericardium*, the heart has a wall made up of three layers: the *myocardium*, *endocardium*, and *epicardium*. Within the heart lie four chambers (two atria and two ventricles) and four valves (two atrioventricular [AV] and two semilunar valves). (See *Inside the heart*.)

Zoom in

Inside the heart

Within the heart lie four chambers (two atria and two ventricles) and four valves (two atrioventricular and two semilunar valves). A system of blood vessels carries blood to and from the heart.

Pericardium

The *pericardium* is a fibroserous sac that surrounds the heart and the roots of the *great vessels* (those vessels that enter and leave the heart). It consists of the fibrous pericardium and the serous pericardium.

Fibrous fits freely

The *fibrous pericardium*, composed of tough, white fibrous tissue, fits loosely around the heart, protecting it.

Serous is smooth

The *serous pericardium*, the thin, smooth inner portion, has two layers:
• The *parietal layer* lines the inside of the fibrous pericardium.
• The *visceral layer* adheres to the surface of the heart.

The space between

Between the fibrous and serous pericardium is the *pericardial space*. This space contains *pericardial fluid* that lubricates the surfaces of the space and allows the heart to move easily during contraction.

I'm supported and protected by a tough, fibrous sac, but I stay comfortable because it has a smooth inner lining.

The wall

The wall of the heart consists of three layers:

The *epicardium*, the outer layer (and the visceral layer of the serous pericardium), is made up of squamous epithelial cells overlying connective tissue.

The *myocardium*, the middle layer, forms most of the heart wall. It has striated muscle fibers that cause the heart to contract.

The *endocardium*, the heart's inner layer, consists of endothelial tissue with small blood vessels and bundles of smooth muscle.

The chambers

The heart contains four hollow chambers: two atria (singular: atrium) and two ventricles.

Upstairs...

The *atria*, the upper chambers, are separated by the *interatrial septum*. They receive blood returning to the heart and pump blood to the ventricles.

...where the blood comes in

The *right atrium* receives blood from the *superior* and *inferior venae cavae*. The *left atrium*, which is smaller but has thicker walls than the right atrium, forms the uppermost part of the heart's left border. It receives blood from the two pulmonary veins.

Downstairs...

The *right* and *left ventricles*, separated by the *interventricular septum*, make up the two lower chambers. The ventricles receive blood from the atria. Composed of highly developed musculature, the ventricles are larger and have thicker walls than the atria.

...where the blood goes out

The right ventricle pumps blood to the lungs. The left ventricle, which is larger than the right, pumps blood through all other vessels of the body.

At rest, only about 20% of my blood goes to skeletal muscles. When I exercise, that percentage can increase to 70%.

The valves

The heart contains four valves, two *AV valves* and two *semilunar valves*.

One way only

The valves allow forward flow of blood through the heart and prevent backward flow. They open and close in response to pressure changes caused by ventricular contraction and blood ejection.

The two AV valves separate the atria from the ventricles. The right AV valve, called the *tricuspid valve*, prevents backflow from the right ventricle into the right atrium. The left AV valve, called the *mitral valve*, prevents backflow from the left ventricle into the left atrium.

One of the two semilunar valves is the *pulmonic valve*, which prevents backflow from the pulmonary artery into the right ventricle. The other semilunar valve is the *aortic valve*, which prevents backflow from the aorta into the left ventricle.

Memory jogger

If you can remember that there are two distinct heart sounds, you can recall that there are two sets of heart valves. Closure of the atrioventricular valves makes the first heart sound, the *lub;* closure of the semilunar valves makes the second heart sound, the *dub.*

On the cusps

The tricuspid valve has three triangular *cusps*, or leaflets. The mitral valve, also called the *bicuspid valve*, contains two cusps, a large anterior and a smaller posterior. *Chordae tendineae* attach the cusps of the AV valves to papillary muscles in the ventricles. The semilunar valves have three cusps that are shaped like half-moons.

Specialized pacemaker cells in my myocardium allow electrical impulse conduction.

Conduction system

Contraction of the heart, occurring as a result of its *conduction system*, causes blood to move throughout the body. (See *Cardiac conduction system,* page 130.)

Setting the pace

The conduction system of the heart contains *pacemaker cells*, which have three unique characteristics:
• *automaticity,* the ability to generate an electrical impulse automatically
• *conductivity,* the ability to pass the impulse to the next cell
• *contractility,* the ability to shorten the fibers in the heart when receiving the impulse.

Feeling impulsive

The *sinoatrial (SA) node,* located on the *endocardial surface* of the right atrium, near the superior vena cava, is the normal pacemaker of the heart, generating an impulse between 60 and 100 times per minute. The firing of the SA node spreads an impulse throughout the right and left atria, resulting in *atrial contraction.*

My conduction system has two backup impulse generators.

Fill 'er up

The *AV node,* situated low in the *septal wall* of the right atrium, slows impulse conduction between the atria and ventricles. This "resistor" node allows time for the contracting atria to fill the ventricles with blood before the lower chambers contract.

Spreading the word — "contract"

From the AV node, the impulse travels to the *bundle of His* (modified muscle fibers), branching off to the right and left bundles. Finally, the impulse travels to the *Pur-*

Zoom in

Cardiac conduction system

Specialized fibers propagate electrical impulses throughout the heart's cells, causing the heart to contract. This illustration shows the elements of the cardiac conduction system.

Interatrial tract

Sinoatrial node

Atrioventricular node

Right bundle branch

Internodal tracts

Bundle of His (atrioventricular bundle)

Left bundle branch

Purkinje fibers

> Electrical impulses help me conduct myself at a special rhythm.

kinje fibers, the distal portions of the left and right bundle branches. These fibers fan across the surface of the ventricles from the endocardium to the myocardium. As the impulse spreads, it brings "the word" to the blood-filled ventricles to contract.

Foolproof

The conduction system has two built-in safety mechanisms. If the SA node fails to fire, the AV node will generate an impulse between 40 and 60 times per minute. If the SA node and AV node fail, the ventricles can generate their own impulse between 20 and 40 times per minute.

Cardiac cycle

The *cardiac cycle* is the period from the beginning of one heartbeat to the beginning of the next. During this cycle, electrical and mechanical events must occur in the proper sequence and to the proper degree to provide adequate blood flow to all body parts. The cardiac cycle has two phases: *systole* and *diastole*. (See *Events in the cardiac cycle*, page 132.)

Contract...

At the beginning of *systole*, the ventricles contract. Increasing blood pressure in the ventricles forces the AV valves (mitral and tricuspid) to close and the semilunar valves (pulmonic and aortic) to open.

As the ventricles contract, ventricular blood pressure builds until it exceeds the pressure in the pulmonary artery and the aorta. Then the semilunar valves open, and the ventricles eject blood into the aorta and the pulmonary artery.

...and release

When the ventricles empty and relax, ventricular pressure falls below the pressure in the pulmonary artery and the aorta. At the beginning of *diastole*, the semilunar valves close to prevent the backflow of blood into the ventricles, and the mitral and tricuspid valves open, allowing blood to flow into the ventricles from the atria.

When the ventricles become full, near the end of this phase, the atria contract to send the remaining blood to the ventricles. Then a new cardiac cycle begins as the heart enters systole again.

The autonomic nervous system increases or decreases my heart activity to meet the metabolic needs of my body. Whew!

The specs for this cycle's engine

Cardiac output refers to the amount of blood the heart pumps in 1 minute. It's equal to the heart rate multiplied by the *stroke volume*, the amount of blood ejected with each heartbeat. Stroke volume, in turn, depends on three major factors: *preload*, *contractility*, and *afterload*. (See *Understanding preload, contractility, and afterload*, page 133.)

Now I get it!

Events in the cardiac cycle

The cardiac cycle consists of the following five events.

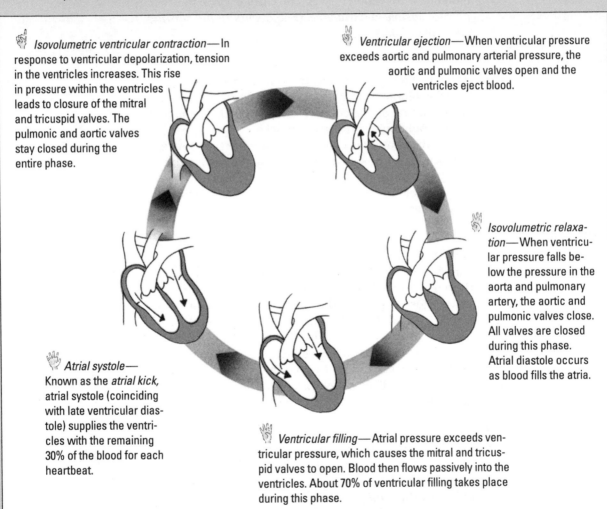

Isovolumetric ventricular contraction—In response to ventricular depolarization, tension in the ventricles increases. This rise in pressure within the ventricles leads to closure of the mitral and tricuspid valves. The pulmonic and aortic valves stay closed during the entire phase.

Ventricular ejection—When ventricular pressure exceeds aortic and pulmonary arterial pressure, the aortic and pulmonic valves open and the ventricles eject blood.

Isovolumetric relaxation—When ventricular pressure falls below the pressure in the aorta and pulmonary artery, the aortic and pulmonic valves close. All valves are closed during this phase. Atrial diastole occurs as blood fills the atria.

Atrial systole—Known as the *atrial kick,* atrial systole (coinciding with late ventricular diastole) supplies the ventricles with the remaining 30% of the blood for each heartbeat.

Ventricular filling—Atrial pressure exceeds ventricular pressure, which causes the mitral and tricuspid valves to open. Blood then flows passively into the ventricles. About 70% of ventricular filling takes place during this phase.

Now I get it!

Understanding preload, contractility, and afterload

If you think of the heart as a balloon, it will help you understand stroke volume.

Blowing up the balloon

Preload is the stretching of muscle fibers in the ventricles. This stretching results from blood volume in the ventricles at end-diastole. According to *Starling's law,* the more the heart muscles stretch during diastole, the more forcefully they contract during systole. Think of preload as the balloon stretching as air is blown into it. The more air the greater the stretch.

The balloon's stretch

Contractility refers to the inherent ability of the myocardium to contract normally. Contractility is influenced by preload. The greater the stretch the more forceful the contraction—or, the more air in the balloon, the greater the stretch, and the farther the balloon will fly when air is allowed to expel.

The knot that ties the balloon

Afterload refers to the pressure that the ventricular muscles must generate to overcome the higher pressure in the aorta to get the blood out of the heart. *Resistance* is the knot on the end of the balloon, which the balloon has to work against to get the air out.

Blood flow

As blood makes its way through the vascular system, it travels through five distinct types of blood vessels, involving three methods of circulation.

Blood vessels

The five types of blood vessels are arteries, arterioles, capillaries, venules, and veins. The structure of each type of vessel differs according to its function in the cardiovascular system and the pressure exerted by the volume of blood at various sites within the system.

Through thick...

Arteries have thick, muscular walls to accommodate the flow of blood at high speeds and pressures. *Arterioles* have thinner walls than arteries. They constrict or dilate to control blood flow to the *capillaries*, which (being microscopic) have walls composed of only a single layer of endothelial cells.

...and thin

Venules gather blood from the capillaries; their walls are thinner than those of arterioles. *Veins* have thinner walls than arteries but have larger diameters because of the low blood pressures of venous return to the heart.

Taking the long way home

About 60,000 miles of arteries, arterioles, capillaries, venules, and veins keep blood circulating to and from every functioning cell in the body. (See *Major blood vessels.*)

Circulation

There are three methods of circulation that carry blood throughout the body: *pulmonary*, *systemic*, and *coronary*.

Pulmonary circulation

Blood travels to the lungs to pick up oxygen and release carbon dioxide.

Returns and exchanges

As the blood moves from the heart, to the lungs, and back again, it proceeds as follows:
• Unoxygenated blood travels from the right ventricle through the pulmonic valve into the *pulmonary arteries*.
• Blood passes through progressively smaller arteries and arterioles into the capillaries of the lungs.
• Blood reaches the *alveoli* and exchanges carbon dioxide for oxygen.
• Oxygenated blood then returns via venules and veins to the *pulmonary veins*, which carry it back to the heart's left atrium.

Body shop

Major blood vessels

This illustration shows the body's major arteries and veins.

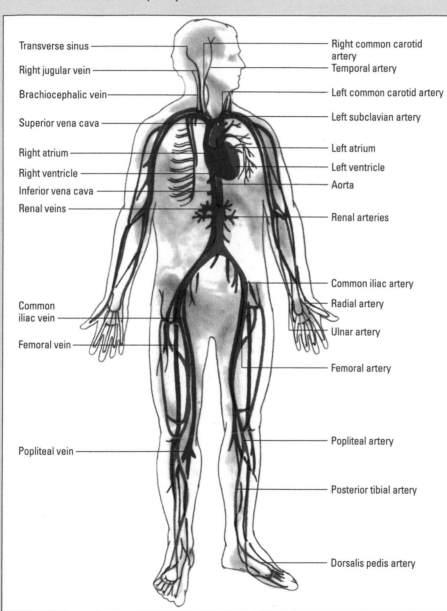

Transverse sinus

Right jugular vein

Brachiocephalic vein

Superior vena cava

Right atrium

Right ventricle

Inferior vena cava

Renal veins

Common iliac vein

Femoral vein

Popliteal vein

Right common carotid artery

Temporal artery

Left common carotid artery

Left subclavian artery

Left atrium

Left ventricle

Aorta

Renal arteries

Common iliac artery

Radial artery

Ulnar artery

Femoral artery

Popliteal artery

Posterior tibial artery

Dorsalis pedis artery

The human body has nearly 60,000 miles of blood vessels. That's enough to circle the globe 2½ times!

Systemic circulation

Blood pumped from the left ventricle carries oxygen and other nutrients to body cells and transports waste products for excretion.

Branching out

The major artery, the *aorta*, branches into vessels that supply specific organs and areas of the body. As it arches out of the top of the heart and down to the abdomen, three arteries branch off the top of the arch to supply the upper body with blood:

- The *left common carotid artery* supplies blood to the brain.
- The *left subclavian artery* supplies the arms.
- The *innominate artery* supplies the upper chest.

As the aorta descends through the thorax and abdomen, its branches supply the organs of the GI and genitourinary systems, spinal column, and lower chest and abdominal muscles. Then the aorta divides into the *iliac arteries*, which further divide into *femoral arteries*.

Division = addition = perfusion

As the arteries divide into smaller units, the number of vessels increases dramatically, thereby increasing the area of tissue to which blood flows, also called the *area of perfusion*.

Dilation is another part of the equation

At the end of the arterioles and the beginning of the capillaries, strong *sphincters* control blood flow into the tissues. These sphincters dilate to permit more flow when needed, close to shunt blood to other areas, or constrict to increase blood pressure.

A large area of low pressure

Although the *capillary bed* contains the smallest vessels, it supplies blood to the largest number of cells. Capillary pressure is extremely low to allow for the exchange of nutrients, oxygen, and carbon dioxide with body cells. From the capillaries, blood flows into venules and, eventually, into veins.

My pumping action can be felt at certain sites. This regular expansion and contraction of arteries is called the *pulse*.

No backflow

Valves in the veins prevent blood backflow. Pooled blood in each valved segment is moved toward the heart by pressure from the moving volume of blood from below. The veins merge until they form two main branches, the *superior vena cava* and *inferior vena cava*, that return blood to the right atrium.

Coronary circulation

The heart relies on the coronary arteries and their branches for its supply of oxygenated blood and depends on the cardiac veins to remove oxygen-depleted blood. (See *Vessels that supply the heart*, page 138.)

The heart gets its part

During left ventricular systole, blood is ejected into the aorta. During diastole, blood flows out of the heart and then through the coronary arteries to nourish the heart muscle.

From the right...

The *right coronary artery* supplies blood to the right atrium, part of the left atrium, most of the right ventricle, and the inferior part of the left ventricle.

...and from the left

The *left coronary artery*, which splits into the *anterior descending artery* and *circumflex artery*, supplies blood to the left atrium, most of the left ventricle, and most of the interventricular septum.

Superficially speaking

The *cardiac veins* lie superficial to the arteries. The largest vein, the *coronary sinus*, opens into the right atrium. Most of the major cardiac veins empty into the coronary sinus, except for the *anterior cardiac veins*, which empty into the right atrium. (See *Cardiovascular changes with aging*, page 139.)

Like any other muscle, I also need oxygen to function. Ah, there's nothing like a little fresh air!

Zoom in

Vessels that supply the heart

Coronary circulation involves the arterial system of blood vessels that supply oxygenated blood to the heart and the venous system that removes oxygen-depleted blood from it.

Anterior view

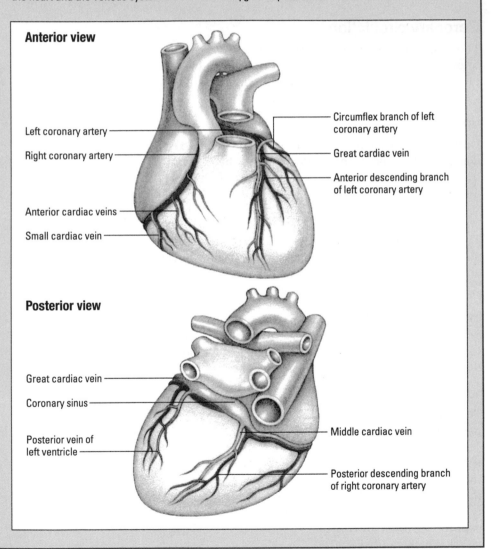

Left coronary artery

Right coronary artery

Anterior cardiac veins

Small cardiac vein

Circumflex branch of left coronary artery

Great cardiac vein

Anterior descending branch of left coronary artery

Posterior view

Great cardiac vein

Coronary sinus

Posterior vein of left ventricle

Middle cardiac vein

Posterior descending branch of right coronary artery

Senior moment

Cardiovascular changes with aging

As a normal part of aging, the heart usually becomes slightly smaller. Contractile strength also declines, making the heart less efficient. In most people, resting cardiac output diminishes 30% to 35% by age 70.

Veins dilate and stretch with age, and coronary artery blood flow drops 35% between ages 20 and 60. The aorta becomes more rigid, causing systolic blood pressure to rise disproportionately higher than the diastolic, resulting in a widened pulse pressure.

Between ages 30 and 80, the left ventricular wall grows 25% thicker from its increased efforts to pump blood. Heart valves also become thicker from fibrotic and sclerotic changes. This can prevent the valves from closing completely, causing systolic murmurs.

Quick quiz

1. During systole the ventricles contract. This causes:
  A. all four heart valves to close.
  B. the AV valves to close and the semilunar valves to open.
  C. the AV valves to open and the semilunar valves to close.
  D. all four heart valves to open.

Answer: B. During systole, the pressure is greater in the ventricles than in the atria, causing the AV valves (the tricuspid and mitral valves) to close. The pressure in the ventricles is also greater than the pressure in the aorta and pulmonary artery, forcing the semilunar valves (the pulmonic and aortic valves) to open.

2. The normal pacemaker of the heart is:
  A. the SA node.
  B. the AV node.
  C. the ventricles.
  D. the Purkinje fibers.

Answer: A. The SA node is the normal pacemaker of the heart, generating impulses 60 to 100 times per minute. The AV node is the secondary pacemaker of the heart (generating 40 to 60 beats per minute). The ventricles are the last line of defense (generating 20 to 40 beats per minute).

3. The pressure the ventricular muscle must generate to overcome the higher pressure in the aorta refers to:
   A.   contractility.
   B.   preload.
   C.   blood pressure.
   D.   afterload.

Answer: D. Afterload is the pressure the ventricular muscle must generate to overcome the higher pressure in the aorta to get the blood out of the heart.

4. The vessels that carry oxygenated blood back to the heart and left atrium are:
   A.   capillaries.
   B.   pulmonary veins.
   C.   pulmonary arteries.
   D.   superior and inferior venae cavae.

Answer: B. Oxygenated blood returns by way of venules and veins to the pulmonary veins, which carry it back to the heart's left atrium.

5. The layer of the heart responsible for contraction is the:
   A.   myocardium.
   B.   pericardium.
   C.   endocardium.
   D.   epicardium.

Answer: A. The myocardium has striated muscle fibers that cause the heart to contract.

Scoring

☆☆☆   If you've answered all five questions correctly, marvelous! You've gotten to the heart of the cardiovascular system.

☆☆   If you've answered four questions correctly, great! We won't call you "vein" if you're a little proud of yourself.

☆   If you've answered fewer than four questions correctly, take heart! It's time to circulate on to the next chapter.

Hematologic system

9

Just the facts

In this chapter, you'll learn:

♦ the way in which blood cells develop

♦ functions of the different blood components

♦ the way in which blood cells clot

♦ blood groups and their significance.

A look at the hematologic system

The hematologic system consists of the blood and bone marrow. Blood delivers oxygen and nutrients to all tissues, removes wastes, and transports gases, blood cells, immune cells, and hormones throughout the body.

Living up to their potential

The hematologic system manufactures new blood cells through a process called *hematopoiesis. Multipotential stem cells* in bone marrow give rise to five distinct cell types, called *unipotential stem cells*. Unipotential cells differentiate into one of the following four types of blood cells:

• erythrocyte
• granulocyte
• agranulocyte
• platelet. (See *Tracing blood cell formation*, pages 142 and 143.)

I've got multipotential!

(Text continues on page 144.)

Now I get it!

Tracing blood cell formation

Blood cells form and develop in the bone marrow by a process called *hematopoiesis*. This chart breaks down the process from when the five unipotential stem cells are "born" from the multipotential stem cell until they each reach "adulthood" as fully formed cells—either erythrocytes, granulocytes, agranulocytes, or platelets.

Multipotential stem cell	Bone marrow		
Unipotential stem cell	Proerythroblast	Early normoblast	Intermediate normoblast
Unipotential stem cell	Myeloblast	Promyelocyte	Neutrophil myelocyte / Eosinophil myelocyte / Basophil myelocyte
Unipotential stem cell	Lymphoblast		Prolymphocyte
Unipotential stem cell	Monoblast		Promonocyte
Unipotential stem cell	Megakaryoblast		Megakaryocyte

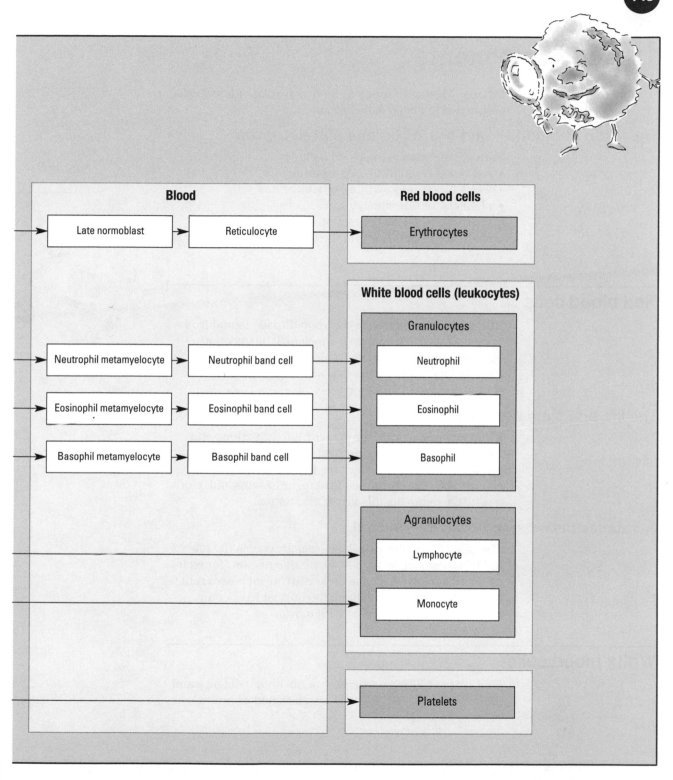

Blood

Late normoblast → Reticulocyte

Neutrophil metamyelocyte → Neutrophil band cell

Eosinophil metamyelocyte → Eosinophil band cell

Basophil metamyelocyte → Basophil band cell

Red blood cells

Erythrocytes

White blood cells (leukocytes)

Granulocytes

Neutrophil

Eosinophil

Basophil

Agranulocytes

Lymphocyte

Monocyte

Platelets

Blood components

Blood consists of various formed elements, or *blood cells*, suspended in a fluid called *plasma*.

The RBCs of blood — and the WBCs and platelets, too

Formed elements in the blood include:
- red blood cells (RBCs), or erythrocytes
- white blood cells (WBCs), or leukocytes
- platelets, or thrombocytes.

RBCs and platelets function entirely within blood vessels; WBCs act mainly in the tissues outside the blood vessels.

The body manufactures billions of new RBCs like me every day!

Red blood cells

RBCs transport oxygen and carbon dioxide to and from body tissues. They contain *hemoglobin*, the oxygen-carrying substance that gives blood its red color. The RBC surface carries *antigens*, which determine a person's *blood group*, or blood type.

The life and times of the RBC

RBCs have an average life span of 120 days. Bone marrow releases RBCs into circulation in immature form as *reticulocytes*. The reticulocytes mature into RBCs in about 1 day. The spleen sequesters, or isolates, old, worn-out RBCs, removing them from circulation.

A balance between removal and renewal

The rate of reticulocyte release usually equals the rate of old RBC removal. When RBC depletion occurs (for example, with hemorrhage), the bone marrow increases reticulocyte production to maintain the normal RBC count. (See *Hematologic changes with aging.*)

White blood cells

Five types of WBCs participate in the body's defense and immune systems. These cells are classified as *granulocytes* or *agranulocytes*.

Senior moment

Hematologic changes with aging

As a person ages, fatty bone marrow replaces some of the body's active blood-forming marrow—first in the long bones and later in the flat bones. The altered bone marrow can't increase erythrocyte production as readily in response to such stimuli as hormones, anoxia, hemorrhage, and hemolysis. Vitamin B_{12} absorption may also diminish with age, resulting in reduced erythrocyte mass and decreased hemoglobin levels and hematocrit.

Granulocytes

Granulocytes include *neutrophils*, *eosinophils*, and *basophils* — collectively known as *polymorphonuclear leukocytes*. All granulocytes contain a single *multilobular nucleus* and *granules* in the cytoplasm. Each cell type exhibits different properties and each is activated by different stimuli.

Swallowing up your enemies

Neutrophils, the most numerous granulocytes, account for 50% to 75% of circulating WBCs. These phagocytic cells engulf, ingest, and digest foreign materials. They leave the bloodstream by passing through the capillary walls into the tissues (a process called *diapedesis)*, then migrate to and accumulate at infection sites.

Making the band

Worn-out neutrophils form the main component of pus. Bone marrow produces their replacements, immature neutrophils called *bands*. In response to infection, bone marrow must produce many immature cells and release them into circulation, elevating the band count.

Allies against allergies

Eosinophils account for 0.3% to 7% of circulating WBCs. These granulocytes also migrate from the bloodstream by diapedesis but do so as a response to an allergic reaction.

Memory jogger

To help yourself remember what neutrophils do, think of two other "**n**" words: **n**umerous and **n**eutralize.

Eosinophils accumulate in loose connective tissue, where they become involved in the ingestion of antigen-antibody complexes.

Fighting the flames

Basophils usually constitute fewer than 2% of circulating WBCs. They possess little or no phagocytic ability. Their cytoplasmic granules secrete *histamine* in response to certain inflammatory and immune stimuli. Histamine makes the blood vessels more permeable and eases the passage of fluids from the capillaries into body tissues.

Agranulocytes

WBCs in the agranulocyte category—*monocytes* and *lymphocytes*—lack specific cytoplasmic granules and have nuclei without lobes. (See *Comparing granulocytes and agranulocytes*.)

We granulocytes serve as the body's first line of cellular defense.

The few and the large

Monocytes, the largest of the WBCs, constitute only 1% to 9% of WBCs in circulation. Like neutrophils, monocytes are phagocytic and enter the tissues by diapedesis. Outside the bloodstream, monocytes enlarge and mature, becoming tissue *macrophages* (also called *histiocytes*).

Protection against infection

As macrophages, monocytes may roam freely through the body when stimulated by inflammation. Usually, they remain immobile, populating most organs and tissues. Collectively, they serve as components of the *reticuloendothelial system*, which defends the body against infection and disposes of cell breakdown products.

Fluid finders

Macrophages concentrate in structures that filter large amounts of body fluid, such as the liver, spleen, and lymph nodes, where they defend against invading organisms. Macrophages are efficient *phagocytes*, cells that ingest microorganisms, cellular debris (including worn-out neutrophils), and necrotic tissue. When mobilized at an infection site, they phagocytize cellular remnants and promote wound healing.

Now I get it!

Comparing granulocytes and agranulocytes

White blood cells (WBCs) are like soldiers fighting off the enemy. Each type of WBC fights a different enemy.

On the front line

Granulocytes, with "platoons" of basophils, neutrophils, and eosinophils, are the first forces "marshalled" against invading foreign organisms.

| Basophils spit histamine at inflammatory and immune stimuli. | Neutrophils eat foreign bodies. | Eosinophils eat antigens and antibodies. |

  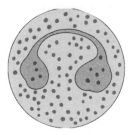

In the trenches

Agranulocytes, with "platoons" of lymphocytes and monocytes, may roam freely on "patrol" when inflammation is reported, but they mainly "dig in" at structures that filter large amounts of fluid (such as the liver) and defend against invaders.

| Lymphocytes eat the enemy, or produce antibodies. | Monocytes eat bacteria, cellular debris, and necrotic tissue. |

Last and, in fact, least (in size)

Lymphocytes, the smallest of the WBCs and the second most numerous (20% to 43%), derive from stem cells in the bone marrow. There are two types of lymphocytes:
• *T lymphocytes* directly attack an infected cell.
• *B lymphocytes* produce antibodies against specific antigens.

Platelets

Platelets are small, colorless, disk-shaped cytoplasmic fragments split from cells in bone marrow called *megakaryocytes.*

These fragments, which have a life span of approximately 10 days, perform three vital functions:
• initiating contraction of damaged blood vessels to minimize blood loss
• forming *hemostatic plugs* in injured blood vessels
• with plasma, providing materials that accelerate blood coagulation.

Blood clotting

Hemostasis is the complex process by which *platelets*, *plasma*, and *coagulation factors* interact to control bleeding.

Stop the bleeding!

When a blood vessel ruptures, local *vasoconstriction* (decrease in the caliber of blood vessels) and *platelet clumping* (aggregation) at the site of the injury initially help prevent hemorrhage. The damaged cells then release tissue factor (thromboplastin), which activates the extrinsic pathway of the coagulation system.

A more long-term solution

However, formation of a more stable clot requires initiation of the complex clotting mechanisms known as the *intrinsic pathway*. This clotting system is activated by a protein, called factor XII, one of 12 substances necessary for coagulation and derived from plasma and tissue.

When cells like me are damaged, we release thromboplastin, which activates the extrinsic portion of the coagulation system.

Come together

The final result of coagulation is a *fibrin clot*, an accumulation of a fibrous, insoluble protein at the site of the injury. (See *How blood clots*, page 150.)

Coagulation factors

The materials that platelets and plasma provide work with *coagulation factors* to serve as *precursor compounds* in the clotting (coagulation) of blood.

12 factors clotting

Designated by name and Roman numeral, these *coagulation factors* are activated in a chain reaction, each one in turn activating the next factor in the chain:
• Factor I, *fibrinogen*, is a high-molecular-weight protein synthesized in the liver and converted to fibrin during the coagulation cascade.
• Factor II, *prothrombin*, is a protein synthesized in the liver in the presence of vitamin K and converted to thrombin during coagulation.
• Factor III, *tissue factor (thromboplastin)*, is released from damaged tissue; it's required to initiate the second phase, the extrinsic pathway.
• Factor IV, consisting of *calcium ions*, is required throughout the entire clotting sequence.
• Factor V, or *labile factor (proaccelerin)*, is a protein that's synthesized in the liver and functions during the common pathway phase of the coagulation system.
• Factor VII, *serum prothrombin conversion accelerator* or *stable factor (proconvertin)*, is a protein synthesized in the liver in the presence of vitamin K; it's activated by Factor III in the extrinsic system.
• Factor VIII, *antihemophilic factor (antihemophilic globulin)*, is a protein synthesized in the liver and required during the intrinsic phase of the coagulation system.
• Factor IX, *plasma thromboplastin component*, a protein synthesized in the liver in the presence of vitamin K, is required in the intrinsic phase of the coagulation system.
• Factor X, *Stuart factor (Stuart-Prower factor)*, is a protein synthesized in the liver in the presence of vitamin

Coagulation factors stimulate clot formation without hindering blood flow.

Now I get it!

How blood clots

When a blood vessel is severed or injured, three interrelated processes take place.

Constriction and aggregation

Immediately, the vessels affected by the injury contract *(constriction)*, reducing blood flow. Also, platelets, stimulated by the exposed collagen of the damaged cells, begin to clump together *(aggregation)*. Aggregation provides a temporary seal and a site for clotting to take place. The platelets release a number of substances that enhance constriction and aggregation.

Clotting pathways

Clotting, or *coagulation*—the transformation of blood from a liquid to a solid—may be initiated through two different pathways, the intrinsic pathway or the extrinsic pathway. The *intrinsic pathway* is activated when plasma comes in contact with damaged vessel surfaces. The *extrinsic pathway* is activated when tissue factor (a substance released by damaged endothelial cells) comes into contact with one of the clotting factors.

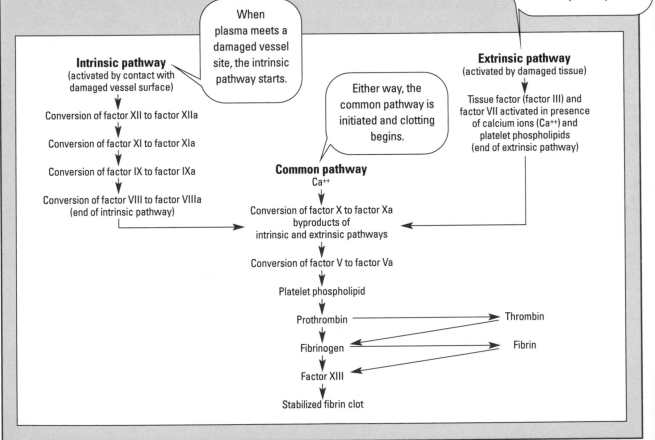

Intrinsic pathway
(activated by contact with damaged vessel surface)

When plasma meets a damaged vessel site, the intrinsic pathway starts.

Conversion of factor XII to factor XIIa

Conversion of factor XI to factor XIa

Conversion of factor IX to factor IXa

Conversion of factor VIII to factor VIIIa
(end of intrinsic pathway)

Either way, the common pathway is initiated and clotting begins.

Common pathway
Ca++

Conversion of factor X to factor Xa
byproducts of
intrinsic and extrinsic pathways

Conversion of factor V to factor Va

Platelet phospholipid

Prothrombin ⟶ Thrombin

Fibrinogen ⟶ Fibrin

Factor XIII

Stabilized fibrin clot

When trauma occurs within a cell, the extrinsic pathway starts.

Extrinsic pathway
(activated by damaged tissue)

Tissue factor (factor III) and factor VII activated in presence of calcium ions (Ca++) and platelet phospholipids
(end of extrinsic pathway)

K; it's required in the common pathway of the coagulation system.
• Factor XI, *plasma thromboplastin antecedent*, is a protein synthesized in the liver and required in the intrinsic pathway.
• Factor XII, *Hageman factor*, is a protein required in the intrinsic pathway.
• Factor XIII, *fibrin stabilizing factor*, is a protein required to stabilize the fibrin strands in the common pathway phase of the coagulation system.

Blood groups

Blood groups are determined by the presence or absence of genetically determined *antigens* or *agglutinogens* (glycoproteins) on the surface of RBCs. A, B, and Rh are the most clinically significant blood antigens.

ABO groups

Testing for the presence of A and B antigens on RBCs is the most important system for classifying blood:
• Type A blood has A antigen on its surface.
• Type B blood has B antigen.
• Type AB blood has both A and B antigens.
• Type O blood has neither A nor B antigen.

Opposites don't attract

Plasma may contain *antibodies* that interact with these antigens, causing the cells to *agglutinate*, or combine into a mass. However, plasma can't contain antibodies to its own cell antigen or it would destroy itself. Thus, type A blood has A antigen but no A antibodies; however, it does have B antibodies.

Making a match

Precise blood-typing and crossmatching (mixing and observing for agglutination of donor cells) are essential, especially for blood transfusions. A donor's blood must be compatible with a recipient's or the result can be fatal. The following blood groups are compatible:
• type A with type A or O
• type B with type B or O

Memory jogger

Blood types are easy to remember because they're named after the antigens they contain—A or B or both A and B—except for type O, which contains neither. The O serves as a nice visual reminder of that absence.

Now I get it!

Reviewing blood type compatibility

Blood typing is an important step before a transfusion.

Precise blood typing and crossmatching can prevent the transfusion of incompatible blood, which can be fatal. Usually, typing the recipient's blood and crossmatching it with available donor blood take less than 1 hour.

Making a match

Agglutinogen (an antigen in red blood cells) and *agglutinin* (an antibody in plasma) distinguish the four ABO blood groups. This chart shows ABO compatibility from the perspectives of the recipient and the donor.

Blood group	Antibodies present in plasma	Compatible RBCs	Compatible plasma
Recipient			
O	Anti-A and anti-B	O	O, A, B, AB
A	Anti-B	A, O	A, AB
B	Anti-A	B, O	B, AB
AB	Neither anti-A nor anti-B	AB, A, B, O	AB
Donor			
O	Anti-A and anti-B	O, A, B, AB	O
A	Anti-B	A, AB	A, O
B	Anti-A	B, AB	B, O
AB	Neither anti-A nor anti-B	AB	AB, A, B, O

- type AB with type A, B, AB, or O
- type O with type O only. (See *Reviewing blood type compatibility*.)

Rh typing

Rh typing determines whether Rh factor is present or absent in blood. Of the eight types of Rh antigens, only C, D, and E are common.

Positive and negative types

Typically, blood contains the Rh antigen. Blood with the Rh antigen is Rh-positive; blood without the Rh antigen is Rh-negative. Anti-Rh antibodies can appear only in a person who has become sensitized. Anti-Rh antibodies can appear in the blood of an Rh-negative person after entry of Rh-positive RBCs in the bloodstream — for example, from transfusion of Rh-positive blood. An Rh-negative female who carries an Rh-positive fetus may also acquire anti-Rh antibodies.

Quick quiz

1. The component of blood that triggers defense and immune responses is the:

    A. WBC.
    B. platelet.
    C. RBC.
    D. hemoglobin.

Answer: A. Because of their phagocytic capabilities, WBCs serve as the body's first line of cellular defense against foreign organisms.

2. The complex process by which platelets, plasma, and coagulation factors interact to control bleeding is called:

    A. phagocytosis.
    B. hematopoiesis.
    C. hemostasis.
    D. diapedesis.

Answer: C. Hemostasis is achieved through a three-part process: vasoconstriction, platelet aggregation, and coagulation.

3. Blood cells form and develop in the:

    A. platelet.
    B. liver.
    C. pancreas.
    D. bone marrow.

Answer: D. Multipotential stem cells in the bone marrow give rise to five distinct cell types called unipotential stem cells. Each of these stem cells can differentiate into an erythrocyte, a granulocyte, an agranulocyte, or a platelet.

4. The most numerous type of granulocytes are the:
   A. bands.
   B. neutrophils.
   C. eosinophils.
   D. basophils.

Answer: B. Neutrophils are the most numerous granulocytes, accounting for 50% to 75% of circulating WBCs.

5. Blood groups are determined by testing for A and B antigens on the:
   A. RBC.
   B. WBC.
   C. leukocyte.
   D. platelet.

Answer: A. Blood groups are determined by the presence or absence of antigens or agglutinogens on the surface of RBCs.

Scoring

☆☆☆   If you answered all five questions correctly, wonderful! You're clearly thinking hemato-logically!

☆☆   If you answered four questions correctly, great. You've coagulated all the information in this chapter into a solid understanding of blood.

☆   If you answered fewer than four questions correctly, be positive (or A positive, or AB positive). Just read the chapter again and give the quiz another go.

Immune system

Just the facts

In this chapter, you'll learn:

♦ organs and tissues that make up the immune system

♦ functions of the immune system

♦ the body's response when the immune system fails.

A look at the immune system

The immune system defends the body against invasion by harmful organisms and chemical toxins.

Lymphoid rules

Organs and tissues of the immune system are referred to as "lymphoid" because they're all involved with the growth, development, and dissemination of lymphocytes, one type of white blood cells (WBCs). (See *Organs and tissues of the immune system*, page 156.)

The immune system has three major components:
- central lymphoid organs and tissue
- peripheral lymphoid organs and tissue
- accessory lymphoid organs and tissue.

Blood relatives

Although the immune system and blood are distinct entities, they're closely related. Their cells share a common origin in the bone marrow, and the immune system uses the bloodstream to transport its "troops" to the site of an invasion.

Body shop

Organs and tissues of the immune system

The immune system includes organs and tissues in which lymphocytes predominate as well as cells that circulate in the blood. This illustration shows central, peripheral, and accessory lymphoid organs and tissue.

Tonsils

Thymus

Lymphatic vessels and blood capillaries

Spleen

Peyer's patches

Appendix

Bone marrow

We're T and B cells, the two major types of lymphocytes.

Central lymphoid organs and tissues

The bone marrow and the thymus each play a role in the development of B cells and T cells—the two major types of *lymphocytes.*

Bone marrow

The *bone marrow* contains stem cells, which can develop into any of several different cell types. Such cells are *multipotential*, meaning they're capable of taking many forms. The cells of the immune system and the blood develop from stem cells in a process called *hematopoiesis*.

To be B or to be T? That is the question...

Soon after their differentiation from other stem cells, some of the cells destined to become immune system cells serve as sources for *lymphocytes;* other cells of this differentiated group develop into *phagocytes* (cells that ingest microorganisms). Those that become lymphocytes are further differentiated to become either *B cells* (which mature in the bone marrow) or *T cells* (which travel to the thymus and mature there).

'Tis better to receive

B cells and T cells are distributed throughout the lymphoid organs, especially the lymph nodes and spleen. T and B lymphocytes have special receptors that respond to specific antigen molecule shapes. In B cells, this receptor is an immunoglobulin, also called an *antibody.* Antibodies attack pathogens or direct other cells, such as phagocytes, to attack for them.

Thymus

In fetuses and infants, the *thymus* is a two-lobed mass of lymphoid tissue that's located over the base of the heart, in the mediastinum. The thymus helps form T lymphocytes for several months after birth. After this time, it has no function in the body's immunity. It gradually undergoes atrophy until only a remnant remains in adults.

Basic training

In the thymus, T cells undergo a process called *T-cell education,* in which the cells are "trained" to recognize other cells from the same body (self cells) and distinguish them from all other cells (nonself cells). There are five types of T cells, each with a specific function:
• memory cells
• lymphokine-producing cells
• cytotoxic T cells
• helper T cells (T_4 cells)
• suppressor T cells (T_8 cells).

I'm a multipotential cell. That means I'm capable of wearing many different hats.

helper   suppressor   killer

Memory jogger

To recall where lymphocytes mature, think, "B in B, and T in T." **B** cells mature in the **B**one marrow and **T** cells mature in the **T**hymus.

Peripheral lymphoid organs and tissues

Peripheral structures of the immune system include the lymph nodes, the lymphatic vessels, and the spleen.

Lymph nodes

The *lymph nodes* are small, oval-shaped structures located along a network of *lymph channels.* Most abundant in the head, neck, axillae, abdomen, pelvis, and groin, lymph nodes help remove and destroy *antigens* (substances capable of triggering an immune response) that circulate in the blood and lymph.

Fully furnished compartments

Each lymph node is enclosed in a fibrous capsule. From this capsule, bands of connective tissue extend into the node and divide it into three compartments:

☝ The *superficial cortex* contains follicles made up predominantly of B cells.

✌ The *deep cortex* and interfollicular areas consist mostly of T cells.

🤟 The *medulla* contains numerous plasma cells that actively secrete *immunoglobulins.*

Lymphatic vessels

Lymph is a clear fluid that bathes the body tissues. It contains a liquid portion, which resembles blood plasma, as well as WBCs (mostly lymphocytes and macrophages) and antigens. Collected from body tissues, lymph seeps into *lymphatic vessels* across the vessels' thin walls. (See *Lymphatic vessels and lymph nodes.*)

Carried into the cavities...

Afferent lymphatic vessels carry lymph into the *subcapsular sinus* (or cavity) of the lymph node. From here, lymph flows through cortical sinuses and smaller radial medullary sinuses. Phagocytic cells in the deep cortex and medullary sinuses attack antigens carried in lymph. The antigens also may be trapped in the follicles of the superficial cortex. These processes essentially clean the lymph.

Memory jogger

Afferent means to **bear** and efferent means to **bring out.** Therefore, it's easy to remember that the afferent lymphatic vessels **bear** lymph into the sinuses and the efferent lymphatic vessels **bring it out.**

Zoom in

Lymphatic vessels and lymph nodes

Lymphatic tissues are connected by a network of thin-walled drainage channels called *lymphatic vessels.* Resembling veins, the afferent lymphatic vessels carry lymph into lymph nodes; lymph slowly filters through the node and is collected into efferent lymphatic vessels.

It can check in but it can't check out
Lymphatic capillaries are located throughout most of the body. Wider than blood capillaries, they permit interstitial fluid to flow into them but not out.

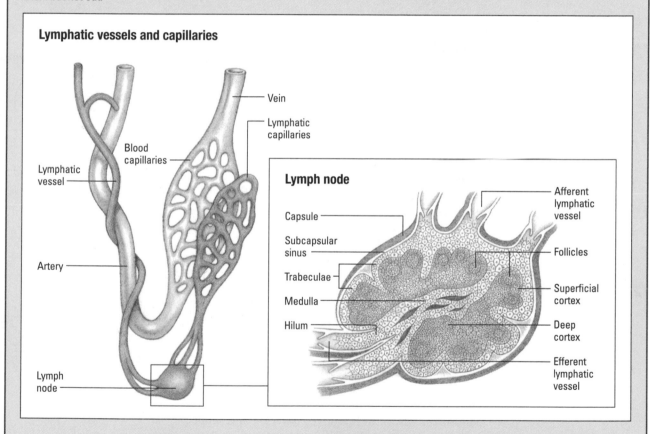

Lymphatic vessels and capillaries

- Vein
- Lymphatic capillaries
- Blood capillaries
- Lymphatic vessel
- Artery
- Lymph node

Lymph node

- Capsule
- Subcapsular sinus
- Trabeculae
- Medulla
- Hilum
- Afferent lymphatic vessel
- Follicles
- Superficial cortex
- Deep cortex
- Efferent lymphatic vessel

...and coming out cleansed

Cleansed lymph leaves the node through *efferent lymphatic vessels* at the *hilum* (a depression at the exit or entrance of the node). These vessels drain into *lymph node chains* that, in turn, empty into large lymph vessels, or trunks, which drain into the subclavian vein of the vascular system.

Getting security clearance

Usually, lymph travels through more than one lymph node because numerous nodes line the lymphatic channels that drain a particular region. For example, axillary nodes (located under the arm) filter drainage from the arms, and femoral nodes (in the inguinal region) filter drainage from the legs. This arrangement prevents organisms that enter peripheral areas from migrating unchallenged to central areas.

Spleen

Located in the left upper quadrant of the abdomen beneath the diaphragm, the *spleen* is a dark red, oval structure that's approximately the size of a fist. Bands of connective tissue from the dense fibrous capsule surrounding the spleen extend into the spleen's interior.

The white and the red

The interior, called the *splenic pulp*, contains white and red pulp. *White pulp* contains compact masses of lymphocytes surrounding branches of the splenic artery. *Red pulp* consists of a network of blood-filled *sinusoids*, supported by a framework of reticular fibers and mononuclear phagocytes, along with some lymphocytes, plasma cells, and monocytes.

A real multitasker

The spleen has several functions:
• Its phagocytes engulf and break down worn-out red blood cells (RBCs), causing the release of hemoglobin, which then breaks down into its components. These phagocytes also selectively retain and destroy damaged or abnormal RBCs and cells with large amounts of abnormal hemoglobin.
• The spleen filters and removes bacteria and other foreign substances that enter the bloodstream; these substances are promptly removed by splenic phagocytes.
• Splenic phagocytes interact with lymphocytes to initiate an immune response.
• The spleen stores blood and 20% to 30% of platelets.

The spleen is the largest lymphatic organ because it must juggle so many tasks.

Accessory lymphoid organs and tissues

The *tonsils*, *adenoids*, *appendix*, and *Peyer's patches* remove foreign debris in much the same way lymph nodes do. They're located in food and air passages — areas in which microbial access is more likely.

Immune system function

Immunity refers to the body's capacity to resist invading organisms and toxins, thereby preventing tissue and organ damage. The immune system is designed to recognize, respond to, and eliminate antigens, including bacteria, fungi, viruses, and parasites. It also preserves the body's internal environment by scavenging dead or damaged cells and patrolling for antigens.

Strategic moves

To perform these functions efficiently, the immune system uses three basic strategies:
- protective surface phenomena
- general host defenses
- specific immune responses.

Protective surface phenomena

Strategically placed physical, chemical, and mechanical barriers work to prevent the entry of potentially harmful organisms.

The forward guard

Intact and healing *skin* and *mucous membranes* provide the first line of defense against microbial invasion, preventing attachment of microorganisms. Skin *desquamation* (normal cell turnover) and low pH further impede bacterial colonization. Seromucous surfaces are protected by antibacterial substances — for instance, the enzyme *lysozyme*, which is found in tears, saliva, and nasal secretions.

Breathe easy...

In the respiratory system (the easiest part of the body for microorganisms to enter), *nasal hairs* and *turbulent airflow* through the nostrils filter out foreign materials.

Nasal secretions contain an immunoglobulin that discourages microbe adherence. Also, a mucous layer, which is continuously sloughed off and replaced, lines the respiratory tract and provides additional protection.

...and swallow

In the GI tract, bacteria are mechanically removed by saliva, swallowing, peristalsis, and defecation. In addition, the low pH of gastric secretions is *bactericidal* (bacteria-killing), rendering the stomach virtually free from live bacteria.

The remainder of the GI system is protected through *colonization resistance*, in which resident bacteria prevent other microorganisms from permanently making a home.

No colonization allowed

The urinary system is sterile except for the distal end of the urethra and the urinary meatus. Urine flow, low urine pH, immunoglobulin and, in men, the bactericidal effects of *prostatic fluid* work together to impede bacterial colonization. A series of sphincters also inhibits bacterial migration.

I'm a resident bacterium. I live in harmony with the body without causing disease, but I keep other microorganisms from colonizing my turf.

General host defenses

When an antigen does penetrate the skin or mucous membrane, the immune system launches nonspecific cellular responses in an effort to identify and remove the invader.

Raising the red flag

The first of the nonspecific responses against an antigen, the *inflammatory response*, involves vascular and cellular changes, including the production and release of such chemical substances as heparin, histamine, and kinin. These changes eliminate dead tissue, microorganisms, toxins, and inert foreign matter. (See *Understanding the inflammatory response.*)

Inflammatory response rousers

Polymorphonuclear leukocytes play a big role in the inflammatory response:
• *Neutrophils*, the most numerous polymorphonuclear leukocyte, increase dramatically in number in response to infection and inflammation. They're the main constitute of pus and are highly mobile. Neutrophils are attracted to ar-

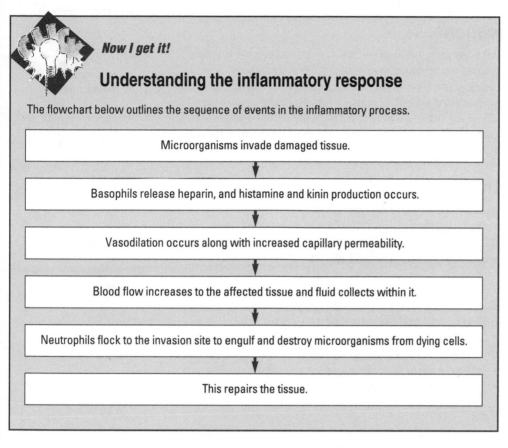

Now I get it!

Understanding the inflammatory response

The flowchart below outlines the sequence of events in the inflammatory process.

| Microorganisms invade damaged tissue. |

↓

| Basophils release heparin, and histamine and kinin production occurs. |

↓

| Vasodilation occurs along with increased capillary permeability. |

↓

| Blood flow increases to the affected tissue and fluid collects within it. |

↓

| Neutrophils flock to the invasion site to engulf and destroy microorganisms from dying cells. |

↓

| This repairs the tissue. |

eas of inflammation. They engulf, digest, and dispose of invading organisms through a process called *phagocytosis*.

• *Eosinophils* multiply in allergic and parasitic disorders. Although their phagocytic function isn't clearly understood, evidence suggests that they participate in host defense against parasites.

• *Basophils* and *mast cells* also function in immune disorders. Basophils circulate in peripheral blood, whereas mast cells accumulate in connective tissue, particularly in the lungs, intestines, and skin. (Mast cells are not blood cells.) Both cells have surface receptors for immunoglobuin (Ig) E. When their receptors are cross-linked by an IgE antigen complex, they release mediators characteristic of the allergic response.

Specific immune responses

All foreign substances elicit the same general host defenses. In addition, particular microorganisms or molecules activate specific immune responses and can involve specialized sets of immune cells. Specific responses, classified as either *humoral immunity* or *cell-mediated immunity*, are produced by lymphocytes (B cells and T cells).

Humoral immunity

In this response, an invading antigen causes B cells to divide and differentiate into plasma cells. Each plasma cell, in turn, produces and secretes large amounts of antigen-specific immunoglobulins into the bloodstream.

The Ig guard

Each of the five types of *immunoglobulins* (IgA, IgD, IgE, IgG, and IgM) serves a particular function:
• IgA, IgG, and IgM guard against viral and bacterial invasion.
• IgD acts as an antigen receptor of B cells.
• IgE causes an allergic response.

"Y?" Because it's our job

Immunoglobulins have a special molecular structure that creates a Y shape. The upper fork of the Y is designed to attach to a particular antigen; the lower stem enables the immunoglobulin to link with other structures in the immune system. Depending on the antigen, immunoglobulins can work in one of several ways:
• They can disable certain bacteria by linking with toxins that the bacteria produce; these immunoglobulins are called *antitoxins*.
• They can *opsonize* (coat) bacteria, making them targets for scavenging by phagocytosis. (See *How macrophages accomplish phagocytosis.*)
• Most commonly, they can link to antigens, causing the immune system to produce and circulate enzymes called *complement*.

A break in the action

After the body's initial exposure to an antigen, a time lag occurs during which little or no antibody can be detected. During this time, the B cell recognizes the antigen and

My job is to produce antibodies. They attack the antigens for me.

I like the direct approach. Sometimes I attack antigens myself.

Now I get it!

How macrophages accomplish phagocytosis

Microorganisms and other antigens that invade the skin and mucous membranes are removed by *phagocytosis,* a defense mechanism carried out by macrophages (mononuclear leukocytes) and neutrophils (polymorphonuclear leukocytes). Here's how macrophages accomplish phagocytosis.

Chemotaxis
Chemotactic factors attract macrophages to the antigen site.

Microorganism

Chemotactic factors

Macrophage

Opsonization
Antibody (immunoglobulin G) or complement fragment coats the microorganism, enhancing macrophage binding to the antigen, now called an *opsinogen.*

Opsonized microorganism

Ingestion
The macrophage extends its membrane around the opsonized microorganism, engulfing it within a vacuole *(phagosome).*

Developing phagosome

Digestion
As the phagosome shifts away from the cell periphery, it merges with lysosomes, forming a *phagolysosome,* where antigen destruction occurs.

Phagolysosome

Release
When digestion is complete, the macrophage expels digestive debris, including lysosomes, prostaglandins, complement components, and interferon, which continue to mediate the immune response.

Digestive debris

the sequence of division, differentiation, and antibody formation begins.

First response

The *primary antibody response* occurs 4 to 10 days after first-time antigen exposure. During this response, immunoglobulin levels increase, then quickly dissipate, and IgM antibodies form.

Second response: Hit 'em hard, hit 'em fast

Subsequent exposure to the same antigen initiates a *secondary antibody response*. In this response, memory B cells manufacture antibodies (now mainly IgG), achieving peak levels in 1 to 2 days. These elevated levels persist for months, then fall slowly. Thus, the secondary antibody response is faster, more intense, and more persistent than the primary response. This response intensifies with each subsequent exposure to the same antigen.

Getting complex

After the antibody reacts to the antigen, an *antigen-antibody complex* forms. The complex serves several functions. First, a macrophage processes the antigen and presents it to antigen-specific B cells. Then the antibody activates the complement system, causing an *enzymatic cascade* that destroys the antigen.

You thought I was slow in the first round? Well, just wait. I always come back faster and meaner in the second.

Complement system

The activated *complement system*, which bridges humoral and cell-mediated immunity, attracts phagocytic neutrophils and macrophages to the antigen site.

Working together

Indispensable to the humoral immune response, the complement system consists of about 25 enzymes that "complement" the work of antibodies by aiding phagocytosis or destroying bacteria cells (through puncture of their cell membranes).

A ripple effect

Complement proteins travel in the bloodstream in an inactive form. When the first complement substance is triggered (typically by an antibody interlocked with an antigen), it sets in motion a ripple effect. As each component is activated in turn, it acts on the next component in a sequence of carefully controlled steps called the *complement cascade*.

Attack mode

This cascade leads to the creation of the *membrane attack complex.* Inserted into the membrane of the target cell, this complex creates a channel through which fluids and molecules flow in and out. The target cell then swells and eventually bursts.

Other benefits flow from the complement cascade

By-products of the complement cascade also produce:
• the inflammatory response (resulting from release of the contents of mast cells and basophils)
• stimulation and attraction of neutrophils (which participate in phagocytosis)
• coating of target cells by C3b (an inactivated fragment of the complement protein C3), making them attractive to phagocytes.

The complement cascade plays a crucial role in the inflammatory response.

Cell-mediated immunity

Cell-mediated immunity protects the body against bacterial, viral, and fungal infections and provides resistance against transplanted cells and tumor cells.

Ever vigilant

In this immune response, a macrophage processes the antigen, which is then presented to T cells. Some T cells become sensitized and destroy the antigen; others release *lymphokines,* which activate macrophages that destroy the antigen. Sensitized T cells then travel through the blood and lymphatic systems, providing ongoing surveillance in their quest for specific antigens.

The great communicators

Cytokines are low-molecular-weight proteins that are involved in the communication between macrophages and lymphocytes. These proteins are responsible for inducing and regulating a variety of immune and inflammatory responses. Cytokines include colony-stimulating factors, interferons, interleukins, tumor necrosis factors, and transforming growth factor.

Immune system malfunction

Because of their complexity, the processes involved in host defense and immune response may malfunction. When the body's defenses are exaggerated, misdirected, or either absent or depressed, the result may be a *hypersensitivity disorder*, *autoimmunity*, or *immunodeficiency*, respectively.

> Hypersensitivity stems from an exaggerated or inappropriate immune response.

Hypersensitivity disorders

An exaggerated or inappropriate immune response may lead to various hypersensitivity disorders.

Typing them out

Such disorders are classified as type I through type IV, depending on which immune system activity causes tissue damage, although some overlap exists:

• Type I disorders are *anaphylactic (immediate, atopic, IgE-mediated reaginic) reactions*. Examples of type I disorders include systemic anaphylaxis, hay fever (seasonal allergic rhinitis), reactions to insect stings, some food and drug reactions, some cases of urticaria, and infantile eczema.

• Type II disorders are *cytotoxic (cytolytic, complement-dependent cytotoxicity) reactions*. Examples of type II disorders include Goodpasture's syndrome, autoimmune hemolytic anemia, transfusion reactions, hemolytic disease of the newborn, myasthenia gravis, and some drug reactions.

• Type III disorders are *immune complex disease reactions*. Examples of type III disorders are reactions associated with such infections as hepatitis B and bacterial endocarditis; cancers, in which a serum sickness-like syndrome may occur; and autoimmune disorders such as systemic lupus erythematosus. This hypersensitivity reaction may also follow drug or serum therapy.

• Type IV disorders are *delayed (cell-mediated) hypersensitivity reactions*. Type IV disorders include tuberculin reactions, contact hypersensitivity, and sarcoidosis.

Autoimmune disorders

Autoimmune disorders are marked by an abnormal response to one's own tissue.

Diffusion can lead to confusion

Autoimmunity leads to a sequence of tissue reactions and damage that may produce diffuse systemic signs and symptoms. Among the autoimmune disorders are rheumatoid arthritis, juvenile rheumatoid arthritis, psoriatic arthritis, ankylosing spondylitis, Sjögren's syndrome, and lupus erythematosus. (See *Immunologic changes with aging.*)

Immunodeficiency

Immunodeficiency disorders are caused by an absent or depressed immune response in various forms.

Unfortunately, no deficiency of immunodeficiency disorders

Immunodeficiency disorders include X-linked infantile hypogammaglobulinemia, common variable immunodeficiency, DiGeorge's syndrome, acquired immunodeficiency syndrome, chronic granulomatous disease, ataxia-telangiectasia, severe combined immunodeficiency disease, and complement deficiencies.

Immunodeficiency disorders occur when the immune system is depressed or on a downward slide.

Senior moment

Immunologic changes with aging

Immune function starts declining at sexual maturity and continues declining with age. During this decline, the immune system begins losing its ability to differentiate between self and nonself, and the incidence of autoimmune disease increases. The immune system also begins losing its ability to recognize and destroy mutant cells, which presumably accounts for the increase in cancer among older people.

Decreased antibody response in older people makes them more susceptible to infection.

Tonsillar atrophy and lymphadenopathy commonly occur.

Total and differential leukocyte counts don't change significantly with age. However, some people over age 65 may exhibit a slight decrease in leukocyte count. When this happens, the number of B cells and total lymphocytes decreases, and T cells decrease in number and become less effective. Also, the sizes of the lymph nodes and spleen reduce slightly.

Quick quiz

1. Stem cells are multipotential and develop into other types of cells through the process of:
    A.   chemotaxis.
    B.   phagocytosis.
    C.   hematopoiesis.
    D.   opsonization.

Answer: C. Hematopoiesis is the formation of blood cells, which occurs in the bone marrow.

2. Cleansed lymph leaves the lymph nodes through:
    A.   afferent lymphatic vessels.
    B.   efferent lymphatic vessels.
    C.   lymphatic capillaries.
    D.   blood capillaries.

Answer: B. Efferent lymphatic vessels drain into lymph node chains, then into large lymph vessels and, finally, into the subclavian vein.

3. During which phase of phagocytosis does a macrophage engulf an opsonized microorganism within a vacuole?
    A.   Chemotaxis
    B.   Opsonization
    C.   Ingestion
    D.   Digestion

Answer: C. During ingestion, the macrophage extends its membrane around the microorganism, engulfing it within a vacuole and forming a phagosome.

Scoring

☆☆☆   If you answered all three questions correctly, impressive! You've responded like a pro to all of our immunologic challenges!

☆☆   If you answered two questions correctly, prodigious! You've proved your multipotential!

☆   If you answered only one question correctly, you might say you have an immunodeficiency. Take some vitamin C, and read this chapter again in the morning!

Hey, want to trade? I'll give you a little oxygen for a bit of carbon dioxide.

Respiratory system

Just the facts

In this chapter, you'll learn:

♦ structures of the respiratory system and their functions

♦ the processes of inspiration and expiration

♦ the way in which gas exchange takes place

♦ problems with the nervous, musculoskeletal, and pulmonary systems that can affect breathing

♦ role of the lungs in acid-base balance.

A look at the respiratory system

The respiratory system consists of the:
- upper respiratory tract
- lower respiratory tract
- lungs and accessory structures
- thoracic cavity.

This system maintains the exchange of oxygen and carbon dioxide in the lungs and tissues. The respiratory system also helps regulate the body's acid-base balance.

Upper respiratory tract

The upper respiratory tract consists primarily of the nose (nostrils and nasal passages), mouth, nasopharynx, oropharynx, laryngopharynx, and larynx. These structures filter, warm, and humidify inspired air. They're also responsible for detecting taste and smell and chewing and swallowing food. (See *Structures of the respiratory system.*)

Nostrils and nasal passages

Air enters the body through the nostrils (*nares*). In the nares, small hairs known as *vibrissae* filter out dust and large foreign particles. Air then passes into the two nasal passages, which are separated by the *septum*. Cartilage forms the anterior walls of the nasal passages; bony structures (*conchae* or *turbinates*) form the posterior walls.

Just passing through

The *conchae* warm and humidify air before it passes into the nasopharynx. Their mucus layer also traps finer foreign particles, which the *cilia* (small, hairlike projections) carry to the pharynx to be swallowed.

Sinuses and nasopharynx

The four paranasal sinuses are located in the frontal, sphenoid, and maxillary bones. The sinuses provide speech resonance.

Air passes from the nasal cavity into the muscular nasopharynx through the *choanae*, a pair of posterior openings in the nasal cavity that remain constantly open.

Oropharynx and laryngopharynx

The oropharynx is the posterior wall of the mouth. It connects the nasopharynx and the laryngopharynx. The laryngopharynx extends to the esophagus and larynx.

Larynx

The larynx contains the vocal cords and connects the pharynx with the trachea. Muscles and cartilage form the walls of the larynx, including the large, shield-shaped thyroid cartilage situated just under the jaw line.

It's nothing to sneeze at. These involuntary defense mechanisms help protect the respiratory system from infection and foreign-body inhalation.

- Sneezing
- Coughing
- Gagging
- Spasms

Body shop

Structures of the respiratory system

This illustration depicts the structures of the respiratory system, which can be divided into the upper and lower respiratory tracts.

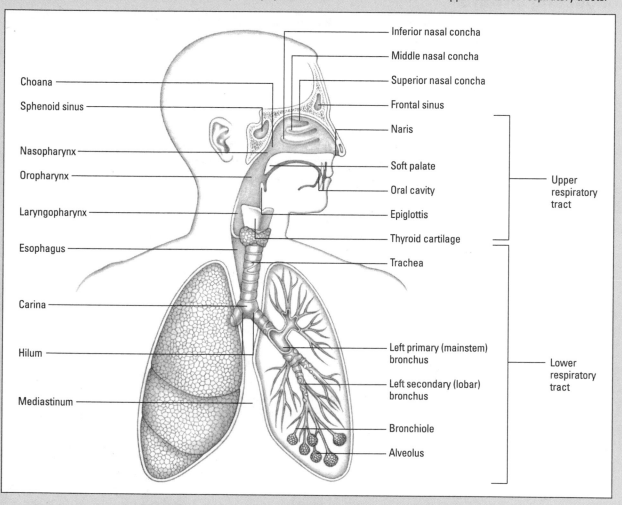

- Choana
- Sphenoid sinus
- Nasopharynx
- Oropharynx
- Laryngopharynx
- Esophagus
- Carina
- Hilum
- Mediastinum

- Inferior nasal concha
- Middle nasal concha
- Superior nasal concha
- Frontal sinus
- Naris
- Soft palate
- Oral cavity
- Epiglottis
- Thyroid cartilage
- Trachea
- Left primary (mainstem) bronchus
- Left secondary (lobar) bronchus
- Bronchiole
- Alveolus

Upper respiratory tract

Lower respiratory tract

Lower respiratory tract

The lower respiratory tract consists of the trachea, bronchi, and lungs. Functionally, the lower tract is subdivided into the *conducting airways* and the *acinus*. The acinus serves as the area of gas exchange. A mucous membrane contains hairlike cilia and lines the lower tract. Cilia constantly clean the tract and carry foreign matter upward for swallowing or expectoration.

Conducting airways

The conducting airways, which contain the trachea and bronchi, distribute air to the respiratory system and, therefore, help facilitate gas exchange.

Trachea

The trachea extends from the *cricoid cartilage* at the top to the carina (also called the *tracheal bifurcation*). The carina is a ridge-shaped structure at the level of the sixth or seventh thoracic vertebra. C-shaped cartilage rings reinforce and protect the trachea to prevent it from collapsing.

Bronchi

The primary bronchi begin at the carina. The right mainstem bronchus — shorter, wider, and more vertical than the left — supplies air to the right lung. The left mainstem bronchus delivers air to the left lung.

Secondary bronchi and the hilum

The mainstem bronchi divide into the five lobar bronchi (secondary bronchi). Along with blood vessels, nerves, and lymphatics, the secondary bronchi enter the pleural cavities and the lungs at the *hilum*. Located behind the heart, the hilum is a slit on the lung's medial surface where the lungs are anchored.

Branching out

Each lobar bronchus enters a lobe in each lung. Within its lobe, each of the lobar bronchi branches into segmental bronchi (tertiary bronchi). The segments continue to branch into smaller and smaller bronchi, finally branching into bronchioles.

The larger bronchi consist of cartilage, smooth muscle, and epithelium. As the bronchi become smaller, they lose cartilage and then smooth muscle. Ultimately, the

Bronchi branch out — from lobar bronchi to segmental bronchi to bronchioles.

smallest bronchioles consist of just a single layer of epithelial cells.

Acinus

Each bronchiole includes terminal bronchioles and the acinus — the chief respiratory unit for gas exchange. (See *A close look at a pulmonary airway*.)

Respiratory bronchioles

Within the acinus, terminal bronchioles branch into yet smaller respiratory bronchioles. The respiratory bronchioles feed directly into alveoli at sites along their walls.

Zoom in

A close look at a pulmonary airway

As illustrated below, each lobule contains terminal bronchioles and the acinus, consisting of respiratory bronchioles and alveolar sacs.

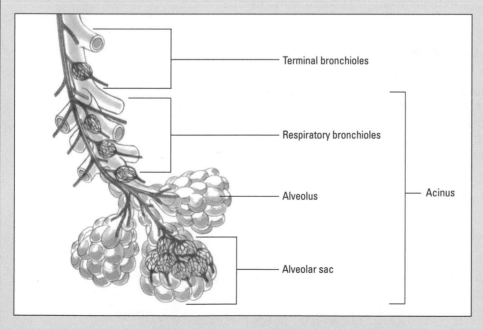

Terminal bronchioles

Respiratory bronchioles

Alveolus

Alveolar sac

Acinus

Alveolar walls contain two basic epithelial cell types:

☝ Type I cells are the most abundant. It is across these thin, flat, squamous cells that gas exchange occurs.

✌ Type II cells secrete *surfactant,* a substance that coats the alveolus and promotes gas exchange by lowering surface tension.

Alveoli

The respiratory bronchioles eventually become alveolar ducts, which terminate in clusters of capillary-swathed alveoli called *alveolar sacs.* Gas exchange takes place through the alveoli.

Lungs and accessory structures

The cone-shaped lungs hang suspended in the right and left pleural cavities, straddling the heart, and anchored by root and pulmonary ligaments. The right lung is shorter, broader, and larger than the left. It has three lobes and handles 55% of gas exchange. The left lung has two lobes. Each lung's concave base rests on the diaphragm; the apex extends about ½″ (1.5 cm) above the first rib.

I hang out in the right and left pleural cavities.

Pleura and pleural cavities

The pleura — the membrane that totally encloses the lung — is composed of a visceral layer and a parietal layer. The visceral pleura hugs the entire lung surface, including the areas between the lobes. The parietal pleura lines the inner surface of the chest wall and upper surface of the diaphragm.

Serous fluid has serious functions

The pleural cavity — the tiny area between the visceral and parietal pleural layers — contains a thin film of serous fluid. This fluid has two functions:

☝ It lubricates the pleural surfaces, which allows them to slide smoothly against each other as the lungs expand and contract.

✌ It creates a bond between the layers that causes the lungs to move with the chest wall during breathing.

Thoracic cavity

The thoracic cavity is the area surrounded by the diaphragm (below), the scalene muscles and fasciae of the neck (above), and the ribs, intercostal muscles, vertebrae, sternum, and ligaments (around the circumference.)

Mediastinum

The space between the lungs is called the *mediastinum*. It contains the:
• heart and pericardium
• thoracic aorta
• pulmonary artery and veins
• venae cavae and azygos veins
• thymus, lymph nodes, and vessels
• trachea, esophagus, and thoracic duct
• vagus, cardiac, and phrenic nerves.

Thoracic cage

The thoracic cage is composed of bone and cartilage. It supports and protects the lungs, allowing them to expand and contract.

Posterior thoracic cage

The vertebral column and 12 pairs of ribs form the posterior portion of the thoracic cage. The ribs form the major portion of the thoracic cage. They extend from the thoracic vertebrae toward the anterior thorax.

Anterior thoracic cage

The anterior thoracic cage consists of the manubrium, sternum, xiphoid process, and ribs. It protects the mediastinal organs that lie between the right and left pleural cavities.

Attached or floating free?

Ribs 1 through 7 attach directly to the sternum; ribs 8 through 10 attach to the cartilage of the preceding rib. The other 2 pairs of ribs are "free-floating" — they don't

The ribs, like the vertebrae, are numbered from top to bottom.

Body shop

Locating lung structures in the thoracic cage

The ribs, vertebrae, and other structures of the thoracic cage act as landmarks that can be used to identify underlying structures.

From an anterior view
• The base of each lung rests at the level of the sixth rib at the midclavicular line and the eighth rib at the midaxillary line.
• The apex of each lung extends about ¾" to 1½" (2 to 4 cm) above the inner aspects of the clavicles.
• The upper lobe of the right lung ends level with the fourth rib at the midclavicular line and with the fifth rib at the midaxillary line.
• The middle lobe of the right lung extends triangularly from the fourth to the sixth rib at the midclavicular line and to the fifth rib at the midaxillary line.
• Because the left lung doesn't have a middle lobe, the upper lobe of the left lung ends level with the fourth rib at the midclavicular line and with the fifth rib at the midaxillary line.

From a posterior view
• The lungs extend from the cervical area to the level of the tenth thoracic vertebra (T10). On deep inspiration, the lungs may descend to T12.
• An imaginary line, stretching from the T3 level along the inferior border of the

Anterior view

Suprasternal notch
Right upper lobe
Sternum
Right middle lobe
Right lower lobe
Xiphoid process
Midsternal line
Right midclavicular line

Manubrium
Clavicle
Left upper lobe
Louis' angle
Fourth rib
Left lower lobe
Sixth rib
Costal angle
Left midclavicular line

Posterior view

Scapula

Left scapular line

Midspinal line

T1
T3
T10
T12
Right scapular line

Locating lung structures in the thoracic cage *(continued)*

scapulae to the fifth rib at the midaxillary line, separates the upper lobes of both lungs.
• The upper lobes are situated above T3; the lower lobes are situated below T3 and extend to the level of T10.
• The diaphragm originates around the ninth or tenth rib.

From a lateral view

The right and left lateral rib cages cover the lobes of the right and left lungs, respectively. Beneath these structures, the lungs extend from just above the clavicles to the level of the eighth rib. The left lateral thorax provides access to two lobes; the right lateral thorax, to three lobes.

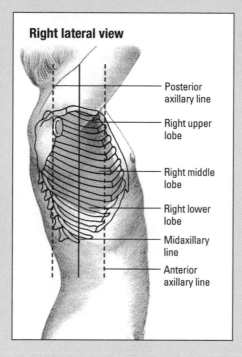

Right lateral view

Posterior axillary line

Right upper lobe

Right middle lobe

Right lower lobe

Midaxillary line

Anterior axillary line

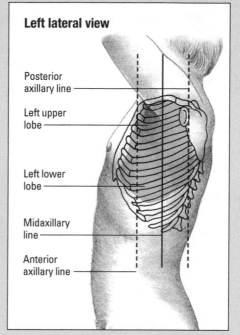

Left lateral view

Posterior axillary line

Left upper lobe

Left lower lobe

Midaxillary line

Anterior axillary line

attach to any part of the anterior thoracic cage. Rib 11 ends anterolaterally, and rib 12 ends laterally.

Bordering on the costal angle

The lower parts of the rib cage (costal margins) near the xiphoid process form the borders of the costal angle — an angle of about 90 degrees in a normal person. (See *Locating lung structures in the thoracic cage.*)

It's suprasternal

Above the anterior thorax is a depression called the suprasternal notch. Because the suprasternal notch isn't covered by the rib cage like the rest of the thorax, the trachea and aortic pulsation can be palpated here. (See *Respiratory changes with aging,* page 180.)

Senior moment

Respiratory changes with aging

As a person ages, the body undergoes respiratory system changes. These changes can include structural changes as well as changes in function.

Structural changes

Age-related anatomic changes in the upper airways include nose enlargement from continued cartilage growth, general atrophy of the tonsils, and tracheal deviations from changes in the aging spine. Possible thoracic changes include increased anteroposterior chest diameter (resulting from altered calcium metabolism) and calcification of costal cartilages, which reduces mobility of the chest wall. Kyphosis advances with age because of such factors as osteoporosis and vertebral collapse.

The lungs become more rigid and the number and size of alveoli decline with age. In addition, a 30% reduction in respiratory fluids heightens the risk of pulmonary infection and mucus plugs.

Pulmonary function changes

Pulmonary function decreases in older people as a result of respiratory muscle degeneration or atrophy. Ventilatory capacity diminishes for several reasons:
- The lungs' diffusing capacity declines; decreased inspiratory and expiratory muscle strength diminishes vital capacity.
- Lung tissue degeneration causes a decrease in the lungs' elastic recoil capability, which results in an elevated residual volume. Thus, aging alone can cause emphysema.
- Closing of some airways produces poor ventilation of the basal areas, resulting in both a decreased surface area for gas exchange and reduced partial pressure of oxygen. The normal partial pressure of oxygen in arterial blood decreases to 70 to 85 mm Hg, and oxygen saturation decreases by 5%.

Inspiration and expiration

Breathing involves two actions: inspiration (an active process) and expiration (a relatively passive process). Both actions rely on respiratory muscle function and the effects of pressure differences in the lungs.

It's perfectly normal!

During normal respiration, the external intercostal muscles aid the diaphragm, the major muscle of respiration. The diaphragm descends to lengthen the chest cavity, while the external intercostal muscles (located between and along the lower borders of the ribs) contract to expand the anteroposterior diameter. This coordinated action causes a reduction in intrapleural pressure, and inspiration occurs. Rising of the diaphragm and relaxation of the intercostal muscles causes an increase in intrapleural pressure, and expiration results. (See *Mechanics of respiration.*)

Body shop

Mechanics of respiration

The muscles of respiration help the chest cavity expand and contract. Pressure differences between atmospheric air and the lungs help produce air movement. These illustrations show the muscles that work together to allow inspiration and expiration.

Anterior view

Scalene muscle

External intercostal muscles

Sternocleidomastoid muscle

Trapezius muscle

Pectoral muscle

Abdominal rectus muscle

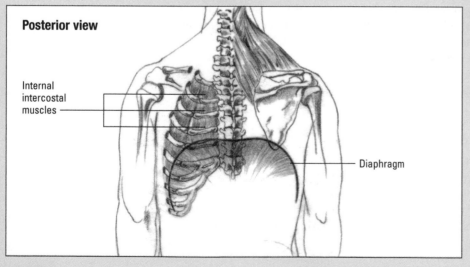

Posterior view

Internal intercostal muscles

Diaphragm

Forced inspiration and active expiration

During exercise, when the body needs increased oxygenation, or in certain disease states that require forced inspiration and active expiration, the accessory muscles of respiration also participate.

Forced inspiration

During forced inspiration:
• the pectoral muscles in the upper chest raise the chest to increase the anteroposterior diameter
• the sternocleidomastoid muscles in the side of the neck raise the sternum
• the scalene muscles in the neck elevate, fix, and expand the upper chest
• the posterior trapezius muscles in the upper back raise the thoracic cage.

Active expiration

During active expiration, the internal intercostal muscles contract to shorten the chest's transverse diameter and the abdominal rectus muscles pull down the lower chest, thus depressing the lower ribs.

Gas station

Oxygen-depleted blood enters the lungs from the pulmonary artery of the heart's right ventricle, then flows through the main pulmonary arteries into the smaller vessels of the pleural cavities and the main bronchi, through the arterioles and, eventually, to the capillary networks in the alveoli. (See *Tracing pulmonary circulation*.) In the alveoli, gas exchange — oxygen and carbon dioxide diffusion — takes place.

When the body's demand for oxygen is increased, such as during exercise, the accessory muscles of respiration help me out.

Internal and external respiration

Effective respiration consists of gas exchange in the lungs, called *external respiration*, and gas exchange in the tissues, called *internal respiration*.

Internal respiration occurs only through diffusion. External respiration occurs through three processes:

ventilation — gas distribution into and out of the pulmonary airways

Now I get it!

Tracing pulmonary circulation

The right and left pulmonary arteries carry deoxygenated blood from the right side of the heart to the lungs. These arteries divide into distal branches, called *arterioles,* which eventually terminate as a concentrated capillary network in the alveoli and alveolar sac, where gas exchange occurs.

Venules — the end branches of the pulmonary veins — collect oxygenated blood from the capillaries and transport it to larger vessels which, in turn, lead to the pulmonary veins. The pulmonary veins enter the left side of the heart and distribute oxygenated blood throughout the body.

💗 *pulmonary perfusion* — blood flow from the right side of the heart, through the pulmonary circulation, and into the left side of the heart

💗 *diffusion* — gas movement through a semipermeable membrane from an area of greater concentration to one of lesser concentration.

Ventilation

Ventilation is the distribution of gases (oxygen and carbon dioxide) into and out of the pulmonary airways. Problems within the nervous, musculoskeletal, and pulmonary systems greatly compromise breathing effectiveness.

Nervous system influence

Involuntary breathing results from stimulation of the respiratory center in the medulla and the pons of the brain. The medulla controls the rate and depth of respiration; the pons moderates the rhythm of the switch from inspiration to expiration.

The central nervous system's respiratory center is located in the lateral medulla.

Musculoskeletal influence

The adult thorax is flexible — its shape can be changed by contracting the chest muscles. The medulla controls ventilation primarily by stimulating contraction of the diaphragm and external intercostal muscles. These actions produce the intrapulmonary pressure changes that cause inspiration.

Pulmonary influence

Airflow distribution can be affected by many factors:
• airflow pattern (see *Comparing airflow patterns*)

Comparing airflow patterns

The pattern of airflow through the respiratory passages affects airway resistance.

Laminar flow
Laminar flow, a linear pattern that occurs at low flow rates, offers minimal resistance. This flow type occurs mainly in the small peripheral airways of the bronchial tree.

Turbulent flow
The eddying pattern of turbulent flow creates friction and increases resistance. Turbulent flow is normal in the trachea and large central bronchi. If the smaller airways become constricted or clogged with secretions, however, turbulent flow may also occur there.

Transitional flow
A mixed pattern known as transitional flow is common at lower flow rates in the larger airways, especially where the airways narrow from obstruction, meet, or branch.

• volume and location of the functional reserve capacity (air retained in the alveoli that prevents their collapse during respiration)
• degree of intrapulmonary resistance
• presence of lung disease.

The path of least resistance

If airflow is disrupted for any reason, airflow distribution follows the path of least resistance.

Increased workload, decreased efficiency

Other musculoskeletal and intrapulmonary factors can affect airflow and, in turn, may affect breathing. For instance, forced breathing (as occurs in emphysema) activates accessory muscles of respiration, which require additional oxygen to work. This results in less efficient ventilation with an increased workload.

Airflow interference and alterations

Other airflow alterations can also increase oxygen and energy demand and cause respiratory muscle fatigue. These conditions include interference with expansion of the lungs or thorax (changes in compliance) and interference with airflow in the tracheobronchial tree (changes in resistance).

Pulmonary perfusion

Pulmonary perfusion refers to blood flow from the right side of the heart, through the pulmonary circulation, and into the left side of the heart. Perfusion aids external respiration. Normal pulmonary blood flow allows alveolar gas exchange, but many factors may interfere with gas transport to the alveoli. Here are some examples:
• Cardiac output less than the average of 5 L/minute decreases gas exchange by reducing blood flow.
• Elevations in pulmonary and systemic resistance reduce blood flow.
• Abnormal or insufficient hemoglobin picks up less oxygen for exchange.

Ventilation-perfusion match

Gravity can affect oxygen and carbon dioxide transport in a positive way. Gravity causes more unoxygenated blood to travel to the lower and middle lung lobes than to the upper lobes.

What happens in ventilation-perfusion mismatch

Ideally, the amount of air in the alveoli (a reflection of ventilation) matches the amount of blood in the capillaries (a reflection of perfusion). This allows gas exchange to proceed smoothly.

This ventilation-perfusion ($\dot{V}/\dot{Q}$) ratio is actually unequal: The alveoli receive air at a rate of approximately 4 L/minute, while the capillaries supply blood at a rate of about 5 L/minute. This creates a $\dot{V}/\dot{Q}$ mismatch of 4:5 or 0.8.

Normal

In the normal lung, ventilation closely matches perfusion.

Dead-space ventilation

Normal ventilation without adequate perfusion usually results from a perfusion defect such as pulmonary embolism.

Shunt

Perfusion without adequate ventilation usually results from airway obstruction, particularly that caused by acute diseases, such as atelectasis and pneumonia.

Silent unit

Inadequate ventilation and perfusion usually stems from multiple causes such as pulmonary embolism with resultant adult respiratory distress syndrome and emphysema.

Blood with CO_2 · Blood with O_2 · Blood with CO_2 and O_2

This explains why ventilation and perfusion differ in the various parts of the lungs. Areas in which perfusion and ventilation are similar have what is referred to as a *ventilation-perfusion match;* in such areas, gas exchange is most efficient. (See *What happens in ventilation-perfusion mismatch.*)

Diffusion

In diffusion, oxygen and carbon dioxide molecules move between the alveoli and capillaries. The direction of movement is always from an area of greater concentration to one of lesser concentration. In the process, oxygen moves across the alveolar and capillary membranes, dissolves in the plasma, and then passes through the red blood cell (RBC) membrane. Carbon dioxide moves in the opposite direction.

The interesting thing about interstitial spaces

The epithelial membranes lining the alveoli and capillaries must be intact. Both the alveolar epithelium and the capillary endothelium are composed of a single layer of cells. Between these layers are tiny interstitial spaces filled with elastin and collagen.

From the RBCs to the alveoli

Normally, oxygen and carbon dioxide move easily through all of these layers. Oxygen moves from the alveoli into the bloodstream, where it's taken up by hemoglobin in the RBCs. When oxygen arrives in the bloodstream, it displaces carbon dioxide (the by-product of metabolism), which diffuses from RBCs into the blood and then to the alveoli.

To bind or not to bind

Most transported oxygen binds with hemoglobin to form oxyhemoglobin; however, a small portion dissolves in the plasma. The portion of oxygen that dissolves in plasma can be measured as the partial pressure of oxygen in arterial blood, or Pao_2.

After oxygen binds to hemoglobin, RBCs travel to the tissues. Through cellular diffusion, internal respiration occurs when RBCs release oxygen and absorb carbon dioxide. The RBCs then transport the carbon dioxide back to the lungs for removal during expiration. (See *Exchanging gases*, page 188.)

During diffusion, oxygen and carbon dioxide travel the same path but in opposite directions.

Move it on over! This is my turf now.

Now I get it!

Exchanging gases

Gas exchange occurs very rapidly in the millions of tiny, thin-membraned alveoli within the respiratory units. Inside these air sacs, oxygen from inhaled air diffuses into the blood while carbon dioxide diffuses from the blood into the air and is exhaled. Blood then circulates throughout the body, delivering oxygen and picking up carbon dioxide. Finally, the blood returns to the lungs to be oxygenated again.

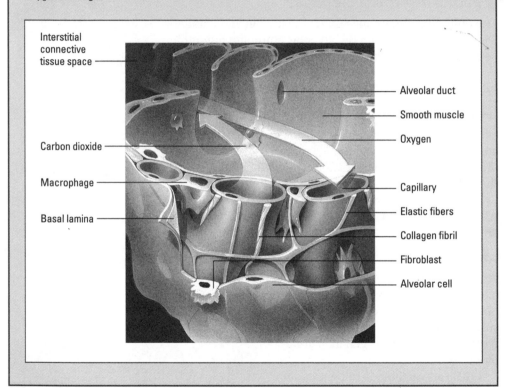

Interstitial connective tissue space

Carbon dioxide

Macrophage

Basal lamina

Alveolar duct

Smooth muscle

Oxygen

Capillary

Elastic fibers

Collagen fibril

Fibroblast

Alveolar cell

Acid-base balance

Oxygen taken up in the lungs is transported to the tissues by the circulatory system, which exchanges it for carbon dioxide produced by metabolism in body cells. Because carbon dioxide is more soluble than oxygen, it dissolves in the blood. In the blood, most of the carbon dioxide forms bicarbonate (base); smaller amounts form carbonic acid (acid).

Respiratory responses

The lungs control bicarbonate levels by converting bicarbonate to carbon dioxide and water for excretion. In response to signals from the medulla, the lungs can change the rate and depth of breathing. This change allows for adjustments in the amount of carbon dioxide lost to help maintain acid-base balance.

It takes cooperation! I send the messages...

Metabolic alkalosis

For example, in *metabolic alkalosis* (a condition resulting from excess bicarbonate retention), the rate and depth of ventilation decrease so that carbon dioxide can be retained; this increases carbonic acid levels.

Metabolic acidosis

In *metabolic acidosis* (a condition resulting from excess acid retention or excess bicarbonate loss), the lungs increase the rate and depth of ventilation to eliminate excess carbon dioxide, thus reducing carbonic acid levels.

Imbalance woes

When the lungs don't function properly, an acid-base imbalance results. For example, they can cause respiratory acidosis through *hypoventilation* (reduced rate and depth of ventilation), which leads to carbon dioxide retention. Conversely, respiratory alkalosis results from *hyperventilation* (increased rate and depth of ventilation), which leads to carbon dioxide elimination.

...and I change the rate and depth of breathing. Together we adjust levels of carbon dioxide and maintain acid-base balance.

Quick quiz

1. Which of the following structures is the chief respiratory unit for gas exchange?
- A. Acinus
- B. Alveoli
- C. Terminal bronchioles
- D. Pulmonary arteries

Answer: A. The acinus is the chief respiratory unit for gas exchange.

2. How many lobes does the right lung have?
   A. Six
   B. Two
   C. Three
   D. One

Answer: C. The right lung has three lobes.

3. During external gas exchange, oxygen and carbon dioxide diffusion occurs in the:
   A. venules.
   B. alveoli.
   C. red blood cells.
   D. body tissues.

Answer: B. Oxygen and carbon dioxide diffusion occurs in the alveoli.

4. When oxygen passes through the alveoli into the bloodstream, it binds with hemoglobin to form:
   A. red blood cells.
   B. carbon dioxide.
   C. nitrogen.
   D. oxyhemoglobin.

Answer: D. When oxygen passes through the alveoli into the bloodstream, it binds with hemoglobin to form oxyhemoglobin.

Scoring

☆☆☆ If you answered all four questions correctly, extraordinary! Take a deep breath! You've responded extremely well to the respiratory system.

☆☆ If you answered three questions correctly, fascinating! You're breezing through these systems like a whirlwind.

☆ If you answered fewer than three questions correctly, get inspired! There are six more quick quizzes to go!

Thanks for studying hard. I can breathe much easier now.

Gastrointestinal system

Just the facts

In this chapter, you'll learn:

♦ two major components of the GI system

♦ phases of digestion

♦ functions of GI hormones

♦ sites and mechanisms of gastric secretions.

A look at the GI system

The GI system has two major components: the *alimentary canal* (also called the *GI tract*) and the *accessory GI organs*.

The GI tract serves two major functions:

digestion, or the breaking down of food and fluid into simple chemicals that can be absorbed into the bloodstream and transported throughout the body

elimination of waste products through excretion of stool.

What goes in must come out. Digestion and excretion are the GI tract's major functions.

Alimentary canal

The alimentary canal is a hollow muscular tube that begins in the mouth and extends to the anus. It includes the pharynx, esophagus, stomach, small intestine, and large intestine. (See *Structures of the GI system*, page 192.) The wall of the alimentary canal is made up of several layers.

Body shop

Structures of the GI system

The GI system includes the alimentary canal (pharynx, esophagus, stomach, and small and large intestines) and the accessory organs (liver, biliary duct system, and pancreas). These structures are illustrated below.

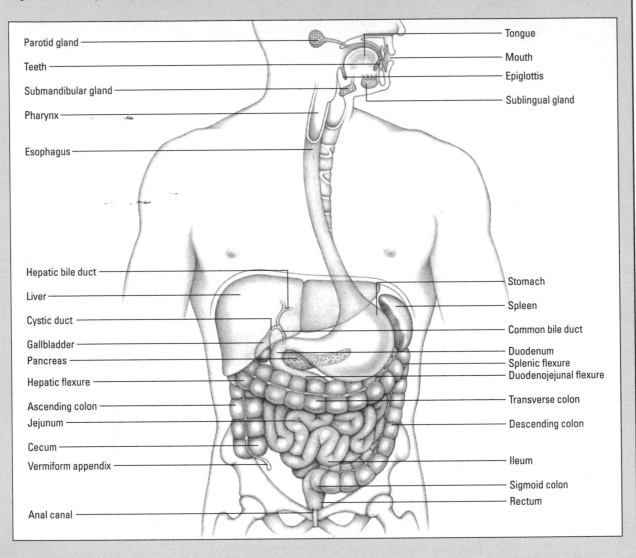

Parotid gland

Teeth

Submandibular gland

Pharynx

Esophagus

Hepatic bile duct

Liver

Cystic duct

Gallbladder

Pancreas

Hepatic flexure

Ascending colon

Jejunum

Cecum

Vermiform appendix

Anal canal

Tongue

Mouth

Epiglottis

Sublingual gland

Stomach

Spleen

Common bile duct

Duodenum

Splenic flexure

Duodenojejunal flexure

Transverse colon

Descending colon

Ileum

Sigmoid colon

Rectum

Mouth

The mouth (also called the *buccal cavity* or *oral cavity*) is bounded by the lips (labia), cheeks, palate (roof of the mouth), and tongue and contains the teeth. Ducts connect the mouth with the three major pairs of salivary glands (parotid, submandibular, sublingual).

These glands secrete saliva to moisten food during chewing. The mouth initiates the mechanical breakdown of food. (See *Oral cavity*, page 194.)

Moisten, chew, and break us down.

Pharynx

The *pharynx* is a cavity that extends from the base of the skull to the esophagus. The pharynx aids swallowing by grasping food and propelling it toward the esophagus.

Esophagus

The *esophagus* is a muscular tube that extends from the pharynx through the mediastinum to the stomach. Swallowing triggers the passage of food from the pharynx to the esophagus. The cricopharyngeal sphincter — a sphincter at the upper border of the esophagus — must relax for food to enter the esophagus. Peristalsis propels liquids and solids through the esophagus into the stomach.

Stomach

The *stomach* is a collapsible, pouchlike structure in the left upper portion of the abdominal cavity, just below the diaphragm. Its upper border attaches to the lower end of the esophagus. The lateral surface of the stomach is called the *greater curvature;* the medial surface, the *lesser curvature.*

Size does matter

The size of the stomach varies with the degree of distention. Overeating can cause marked distention, which pushes on the diaphragm and causes shortness of breath.

Body shop

Oral cavity

The mouth, or oral cavity, is bounded by the lips (labia), cheeks, palate (roof of the mouth), and tongue. The mouth initiates the mechanical breakdown of food.

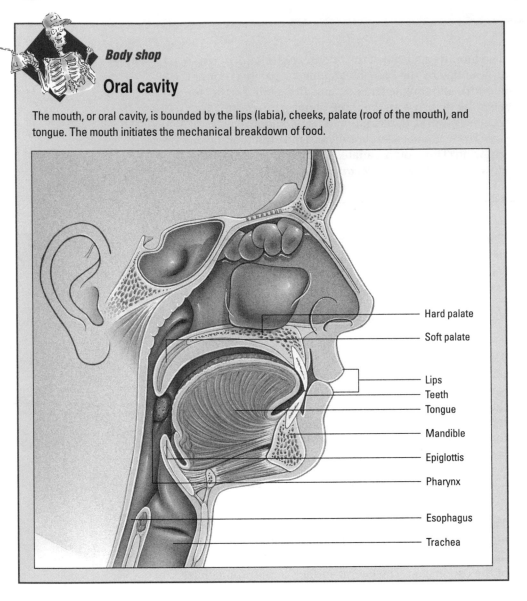

- Hard palate
- Soft palate
- Lips
- Teeth
- Tongue
- Mandible
- Epiglottis
- Pharynx
- Esophagus
- Trachea

The Fab Four

The stomach has four main regions:

The *cardia* lies near the junction of the stomach and esophagus.

The *fundus* is an enlarged portion above and to the left of the esophageal opening into the stomach.

The *body* is the middle portion of the stomach.

The *pylorus* is the lower portion, lying near the junction of the stomach and duodenum.

Just passing through

The stomach has several functions, including:
• serving as a temporary storage area for food
• beginning digestion
• breaking down food into *chyme*, a semifluid substance
• moving the gastric contents into the small intestine.

Small intestine

The *small intestine* is a tube that measures about 20′ (6 m) in length. It's the longest organ of the GI tract and has three major divisions:
• The *duodenum* is the shortest and most superior division.
• The *jejunum* is the middle portion.
• The *ileum* is the longest and most inferior portion.
(See *A look at special cells*, page 196.)

Intestinal wall

The intestinal wall has structural features that significantly increase its absorptive surface area. These features include *plicae circulares* — circular folds of the intestinal mucosa, or mucous membrane lining.

Free villi

Villi and microvilli are also intestinal wall features that increase the absorptive area of the intestinal wall. *Villi* are fingerlike projections on the mucosa. *Microvilli* are tiny cytoplasmic projections on the surface of epithelial cells.

Other structures

The small intestine also contains intestinal crypts, Peyer's patches, and Brunner's glands:
• *Intestinal crypts* are simple glands lodged in the grooves separating villi.
• *Peyer's patches* are collections of lymphatic tissue within the submucosa.
• *Brunner's glands* secrete mucus.

Zoom in

A look at special cells

This cross section of the stomach shows the G-cells (which secrete gastrin) in the pyloric glands. The cross section of the duodenum and jejunum show the S-cells (which secrete secretin) in the duodenal and jejunal glands.

Stomach

G-cell in pyloric glands

S-cell in duodenal and jejunal glands

Completing digestion, absorbing food, and controlling the secretion of bile...the small intestine has a lot of work to do!

Functions

Functions of the small intestine include:
• completing food digestion
• absorbing food molecules through its wall into the circulatory system, which then delivers them to body cells
• secreting hormones that help control secretion of bile, pancreatic fluid, and intestinal fluid.

Large intestine

The *large intestine* extends from the ileocecal valve (the valve between the ileum of the small intestine and the first segment of the large intestine) to the anus. It has six segments:

The *cecum*, a saclike structure, makes up the first few inches.

The *ascending colon* rises on the right posterior abdominal wall, then turns sharply under the liver at the hepatic flexure.

The *transverse colon* is situated above the small intestine, passing horizontally across the abdomen and below the liver, stomach, and spleen. At the left colic flexure, also known as the *splenic flexure,* it turns downward.

The *descending colon* starts near the spleen and extends down the left side of the abdomen into the pelvic cavity.

The *sigmoid colon* descends through the pelvic cavity, where it becomes the rectum.

The *rectum*, the last few inches of the large intestine, terminates at the anus.

Functions

The functions of the large intestine include absorbing water, secreting mucus, and eliminating digestive wastes.

GI tract wall structures

The wall of the GI tract consists of several layers. These layers are the mucosa, submucosa, tunica muscularis, and visceral peritoneum.

Mucosa

The *mucosa*, the innermost layer, also called the *tunica mucosa*, consists of epithelial and surface cells and loose connective tissue. *Villi,* fingerlike projections of the mucosa, secrete gastric and protective juices and absorb nutrients.

Past the lips, past the gums...look out, mucosa, here it comes!

Submucosa

The *submucosa*, also called the *tunica submucosa*, encircles the mucosa. It's composed of loose connective tissue, blood and lymphatic vessels, and a nerve network called the *submucosal plexus*, or *Meissner's plexus*.

Tunica muscularis

The *tunica muscularis*, which lies around the submucosa, is composed of skeletal muscle in the mouth, pharynx, and upper esophagus.

Fibers, fibers everywhere

Elsewhere in the tract, the tunica muscularis is made up of longitudinal and circular smooth muscle fibers. During peristalsis, longitudinal fibers shorten the lumen length and circular fibers reduce the lumen diameter. At points along the tract, circular fibers thicken to form sphincters.

Pucker pouches

In the large intestine, these fibers gather into three narrow bands (*taeniae coli*) down the middle of the colon and pucker the intestine into characteristic pouches (*haustra*).

Networking is key

Between the two muscle layers lies another nerve network — the *myenteric plexus*, also known as *Auerbach's plexus*. The stomach wall contains a third muscle layer made up of oblique fibers. (See *Features of the GI tract wall.*)

Visceral peritoneum

The *visceral peritoneum* is the GI tract's outer covering. It covers most of the abdominal organs and lies next to an identical layer, the *parietal peritoneum*, which lines the abdominal cavity.

A double-layered fold

The visceral peritoneum becomes a double-layered fold around the blood vessels, nerves, and lymphatics. It attaches the jejunum and ileum to the posterior abdominal wall to prevent twisting. A similar fold attaches the transverse colon to the posterior abdominal wall.

So many ways of saying one thing! The visceral peritoneum is known as the tunica adventitia in one part of the body and the tunica serosa in another.

Zoom in

Features of the GI tract wall

Several layers — the tunica mucosa, tunica submucosa, and tunica muscularis — form the wall of the GI tract. This illustration depicts the cellular anatomy of the wall, including special features such as the villi, the peritoneum, the muscles, and a nerve network.

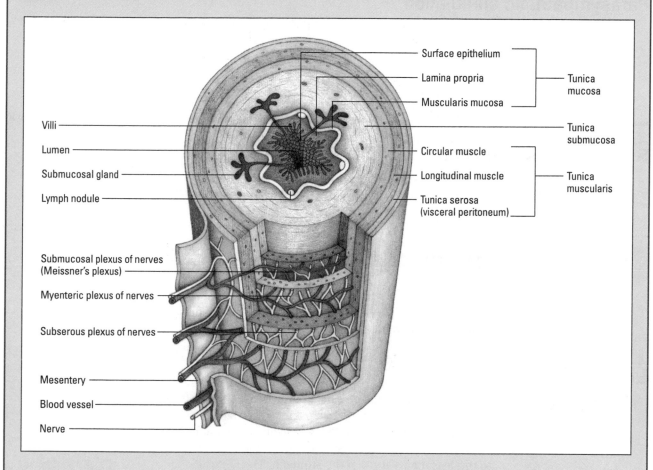

A visceral peritoneum by any other name

The visceral peritoneum has many names. In the esophagus and rectum, it's called the *tunica adventitia;* elsewhere in the GI tract, it's called the *tunica serosa.*

GI tract innervation

Distention of the submucosal plexus stimulates transmission of nerve signals to the smooth muscle, which initiates peristalsis and mixing contractions.

Parasympathetic stimulation

Parasympathetic stimulation of the vagus nerve (for most of the intestines) and the sacral spinal nerves (for the descending colon and rectum) increases gut and sphincter tone. It also increases the frequency, strength, and velocity of smooth-muscle contractions as well as motor and secretory activities.

Sympathetic stimulation

Sympathetic stimulation, by way of the spinal nerves from levels T6 to L2, reduces peristalsis and inhibits GI activity.

Accessory organs of digestion

Accessory organs — the liver, biliary duct system, and pancreas — contribute hormones, enzymes, and bile, which are vital to digestion.

Liver

The body's largest gland, the 3-lb (1.4-kg), highly vascular liver is enclosed in a fibrous capsule in the right upper quadrant of the abdomen. The *lesser omentum*, a fold of peritoneum, covers most of the liver and anchors it to the lesser curvature of the stomach. The *hepatic artery* and *hepatic portal vein*, as well as the common bile duct and hepatic veins, pass through the lesser omentum.

Lobes and lobules

The liver consists of four lobes:
• left lobe

A little respect please! I am the largest gland in the body.

Zoom in

A look at a liver lobule

The liver's functional unit is called a *lobule*. It consists of a plate of hepatic cells, or *hepatocytes,* that encircle a central vein and radiate outward. Separating the hepatocyte plates from each other are *sinusoids,* which serve as the liver's capillary system. Sinusoids carry oxygenated blood from the hepatic artery and nutrient-rich blood from the portal vein.

- right lobe
- caudate lobe (behind the right lobe)
- quadrate lobe (behind the left lobe).

Function...

The liver's functional unit, the *lobule*, consists of a plate of hepatic cells, or *hepatocytes*, that encircle a central vein and radiate outward. Separating the hepatocyte plates from each other are *sinusoids,* the liver's capillary system. Reticuloendothelial macrophages (Kupffer's cells) that line the sinusoids remove bacteria and toxins that have entered the blood through the intestinal capillaries. (See *A look at a liver lobule.*)

...and flow

The sinusoids carry oxygenated blood from the hepatic artery and nutrient-rich blood from the portal vein. Unoxygenated blood leaves through the central vein and flows through hepatic veins to the inferior vena cava.

Ducts

The ducts can be thought of as a subway system that transports bile through the GI tract. *Bile* is a greenish liquid composed of water, cholesterol, bile salts, and phospholipids. It exits through bile ducts (canaliculi) that merge into the right and left hepatic ducts to form the common hepatic duct. This duct joins the cystic duct from the gallbladder to form the common bile duct that leads to the duodenum.

Job description

The liver serves several important functions:
• It plays an important role in carbohydrate metabolism.
• It detoxifies various endogenous and exogenous toxins in plasma.
• It synthesizes plasma proteins, nonessential amino acids, and vitamin A.
• It stores essential nutrients, such as vitamins K, D, and B_{12}, and iron.
• It removes ammonia from body fluids, converting it to urea for excretion in urine.
• It helps regulate blood glucose levels.
• It secretes bile.

Function of bile

Bile has several functions, including:
• emulsifying (breaking down) fat
• promoting intestinal absorption of fatty acids, cholesterol, and other lipids.

When bile salts are MIA

When bile salts are absent from the intestinal tract, lipids are excreted and fat-soluble vitamins are poorly absorbed.

My role in carbohydrate metabolism is very important. I also detoxify toxins in plasma.

Now I get it!

GI hormones: Production and function

When stimulated, GI structures secrete four hormones. Each hormone plays a different role in digestion.

Hormone and production site	Stimulating factor or agent	Function
Gastrin Produced in pyloric antrum and duodenal mucosa	• Pyloric antrum distention • Vagal stimulation • Protein digestion products • Alcohol	Stimulates gastric secretion and motility
Gastric inhibitory peptides Produced in duodenal and jejunal mucosa	• Gastric acid • Fats • Fat digestion products	Inhibits gastric secretion and motility
Secretin Produced in duodenal and jejunal mucosa	• Gastric acid • Fat digestion products • Protein digestion products	Stimulates secretion of bile and alkaline pancreatic fluid
Cholecystokinin Produced in duodenal and jejunal mucosa	• Fat digestion products • Protein digestion products	Stimulates gallbladder contraction and secretion of enzyme-rich pancreatic fluid

Report on bile production

The liver recycles about 80% of bile salts into bile, combining them with bile pigments (biliverdin and bilirubin, the waste products of red blood cell breakdown) and cholesterol. The liver continuously secretes this alkaline bile. Bile production may increase from stimulation of the vagus nerve, release of the hormone secretin, increased blood flow in the liver, and the presence of fat in the intestine. (See *GI hormones: Production and function.*)

Gallbladder

The *gallbladder* is a pear-shaped organ joined to the ventral surface of the liver by the cystic duct. It's covered with visceral peritoneum.

On the job

The gallbladder stores and concentrates bile produced by the liver. It also releases bile into the common bile duct for delivery to the duodenum in response to the contraction and relaxation of Oddi's sphincter.

Pancreas

The *pancreas* is a somewhat flat organ that lies behind the stomach. Its head and neck extend into the curve of the duodenum and its tail lies against the spleen. (See *A look at the gallbladder and pancreas.*) It performs both exocrine and endocrine functions.

Exocrine function

The pancreas's exocrine function involves scattered cells that secrete more than 1,000 ml of digestive enzymes every day. Lobules and lobes of the clusters (*acini*) of enzyme-producing cells release their secretions into ducts that merge into the pancreatic duct.

Endocrine function

The endocrine function of the pancreas is performed by the islets of Langerhans, which are located between the acinar cells.

Alpha, beta...but no omega

There are two types of islet cells: alpha and beta. More than 1 million islets house these two cell types. Beta cells secrete *insulin* to promote carbohydrate metabolism; alpha cells secrete *glucagon*, a hormone that stimulates glycogenolysis in the liver. Both hormones flow directly into the blood. Their release is stimulated by blood glucose levels.

Memory jogger

To remember the difference between exocrine and endocrine, keep in mind that **ex**ocrine refers to **ex**ternal, and **en**docrine refers to **in**ternal.

Body shop

A look at the gallbladder and pancreas

Together, the gallbladder and pancreas constitute the biliary tract. The structures of the biliary tract are depicted in the illustration below.

Right and left hepatic ducts

Cystic duct

Neck of gallbladder

Body of gallbladder

Fundus of gallbladder

Minor duodenal papilla

Sphincter muscles

Major duodenal papilla

Duodenum

Common hepatic duct

Pancreas

Pancreatic duct

Common bile duct

Accessory duct

Superior mesenteric artery and vein

Pancreatic duct

Running the length of the pancreas, the *pancreatic duct* joins the bile duct from the gallbladder before entering the duodenum. Vagal stimulation and release of the hormones secretin and cholecystokinin control the rate and amount of pancreatic secretion.

Digestion and elimination

Digestion starts in the oral cavity, where chewing (*mastication*), salivation (the beginning of starch digestion), and swallowing (*deglutition*) all take place.

When a person swallows, the hypopharyngeal sphincter in the upper esophagus relaxes, allowing food to enter the esophagus. (See *What happens in swallowing*.)

Chewing, salivation, and swallowing. Let digestion begin!

Long day's journey into the stomach

In the esophagus, the glossopharyngeal nerve activates peristalsis, which moves the food down toward the stomach. As food passes through the esophagus, glands in the esophageal mucosal layer secrete mucus, which lubricates the bolus and protects the mucosal membrane from damage caused by poorly chewed foods.

Cephalic phase of digestion

By the time the food bolus is traveling toward the stomach, the *cephalic phase* of digestion has already begun. In this phase, the stomach secretes digestive juices (hydrochloric acid [HCl] and pepsin).

Gastric phase of digestion

When food enters the stomach through the cardiac sphincter, the stomach wall stretches, initiating the gastric phase of digestion. In this phase, distention of the stomach wall stimulates the stomach to release *gastrin*.

Gastrin

Gastrin stimulates the stomach's motor functions and secretion of gastric juice by the gastric glands. Highly acidic (pH of 0.9 to 1.5), these digestive secretions consist mainly of pepsin, HCl, intrinsic factor, and proteolytic enzymes. (See *Sites and mechanisms of gastric secretion*, page 208.)

Now I get it!

What happens in swallowing

Before peristalsis can begin, the neural pattern that initiates swallowing must occur. This process is described here and illustrated below:

• Food pushed to the back of the mouth stimulates swallowing receptor areas that surround the pharyngeal opening.

• These receptor areas transmit impulses to the brain by way of the sensory portions of the trigeminal and glossopharyngeal nerves.

• The brain's swallowing center then relays motor impulses to the esophagus by way of the trigeminal, glossopharyngeal, vagus, and hypoglossal nerves, causing swallowing to occur.

Intestinal phase of digestion

Normally, except for alcohol, little food absorption occurs in the stomach. Peristaltic contractions churn the food into tiny particles and mix it with gastric juices, forming chyme. Next, stronger peristaltic waves move the chyme into the antrum, where it backs up against the

Now I get it!

Sites and mechanisms of gastric secretion

The body of the stomach lies between the lower esophageal, or cardiac, sphincter and the pyloric sphincter. Between these sphincters lie the fundus, body, antrum, and pylorus. These areas have a rich variety of mucosal cells that help the stomach carry out its tasks.

Glands and gastric secretions

Cardiac glands, pyloric glands, and gastric glands secrete 2 to 3 L of gastric juice daily through the stomach's gastric pits. Here are the details:

• Both the *cardiac gland* (near the lower esophageal sphincter [LES]) and the *pyloric gland* (near the pylorus) secrete thin mucus.

• The *gastric gland* (in the body and fundus) secretes hydrochloric acid (HCl), pepsinogen, intrinsic factor, and mucus.

Protection from self-digestion

Specialized cells line the gastric glands, gastric pits, and surface epithelium. Mucous cells in the necks of the gastric glands produce thin mucus. Mucous cells in the surface epithelium produce an alkaline mucus. Both substances lubricate food and protect the stomach from self-digestion by corrosive enzymes.

Other secretions

Argentaffin cells produce gastrin, which stimulates gastric secretion and motility. *Chief cells* produce pepsinogen, which breaks proteins down into polypeptides. Large parietal cells scattered throughout the fundus secrete HCl and intrinsic factor. HCl degrades pepsinogen, maintains acid environment, and inhibits excess bacteria growth. Intrinsic factor promotes vitamin B_{12} absorption in the small intestine.

Stomach structures

- Fundus
- LES
- Body
- Antrum
- Pyloric sphincter
- Pylorus

Gastric mucosa

- Gastric pits
- Mucous surface cell
- Surface epithelium
- Mucous neck cell
- Chief cell
- Parietal cell
- Argentaffin cells
- Gastric glands

pyloric sphincter before being released into the duodenum, triggering the intestinal phase of digestion.

Stomach emptying

The rate of stomach emptying depends on several factors, including gastrin release, neural signals generated when the stomach wall distends, and the *enterogastric reflex*. In this reaction, the duodenum releases secretin and gastric-inhibiting peptide, and the jejunum secretes cholecystokinin — all of which act to decrease gastric motility.

Small intestine

The small intestine performs most of the work of digestion and absorption. (See *Small intestine: How form affects absorption*, pages 210 and 211.)

It only takes a whiff! Digestive juices are secreted in response to smelling, tasting, chewing, or thinking about food.

Small but mighty

In the small intestine, intestinal contractions and various digestive secretions break down carbohydrates, proteins, and fats — actions that enable the intestinal mucosa to absorb these nutrients into the bloodstream (along with water and electrolytes). These nutrients are then available for use by the body.

By the time chyme passes through the small intestine and enters the ascending colon of the large intestine, it has been reduced to mostly indigestible substances.

Large intestine

The food bolus begins its journey through the large intestine where the ileum and cecum join with the ileocecal pouch. Then the bolus moves up the ascending colon and past the right abdominal cavity to the liver's lower border. It crosses horizontally below the liver and stomach, by way of the transverse colon, and descends the left abdominal cavity to the iliac fossa through the descending colon.

Continuing journey of the food bolus

From there, the bolus travels through the sigmoid colon to the lower midline of the abdominal cavity, then to the rectum, and finally to the anal canal. The anus opens to

(Text continues on page 212.)

Now I get it!

Small intestine: How form affects absorption

Nearly all digestion and absorption takes place in the 20′ (6.1 m) of small intestine. The structure of the small intestine, as shown below, is key to digestion and absorption.

Specialized mucosa

Multiple projections of the intestinal mucosa increase the surface area for absorption several hundredfold, as shown in the enlarged views below.

Circular projections *(Kerckring's folds)* are covered by villi. Each villus contains a lymphatic vessel *(lacteal),* a venule, capillaries, an arteriole, nerve fibers, and smooth muscle.

Each villus is densely fringed with about 2,000 microvilli making it resemble a fine brush. The villi are lined with columnar epithelial cells, which dip into the lamina propria between the villi to form intestinal glands *(crypts of Lieberkühn).*

Types of epithelial cells

The type of epithelial cell dictates its function. Mucus-secreting goblet cells are found on and between the villi on the crypt mucosa. In the proximal duodenum, specialized Brunner's glands

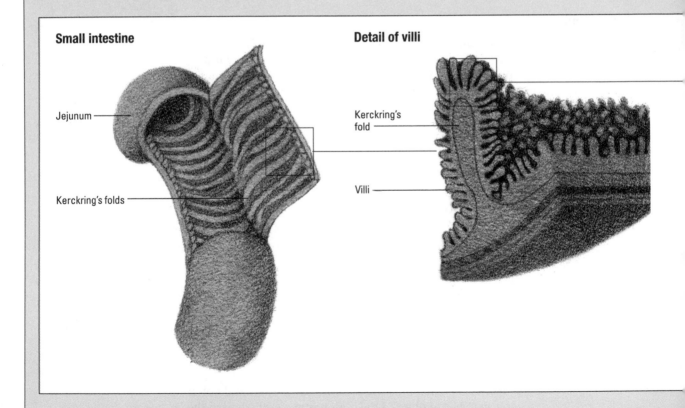

Small intestine

Jejunum

Kerckring's folds

Detail of villi

Kerckring's fold

Villi

also secrete large amounts of mucus to lubricate and protect the duodenum from potentially corrosive acidic chyme and gastric juices.

Duodenal *argentaffin cells* produce the hormones secretin and cholecystokinin. *Undifferentiated cells* deep within the intestinal glands replace the epithelium. *Absorptive cells* consist of large numbers of tightly packed microvilli over a plasma membrane that contains transport mechanisms for absorption and produces enzymes for the final step in digestion.

Intestinal glands

The intestinal glands primarily secrete a watery fluid that bathes the villi with chyme particles. Fluid production results from local irritation of nerve cells and, possibly, from hormonal stimulation by secretin and cholecystokinin. The microvillous brush border secretes various hormones and digestive enzymes that catalyze final nutrient breakdown.

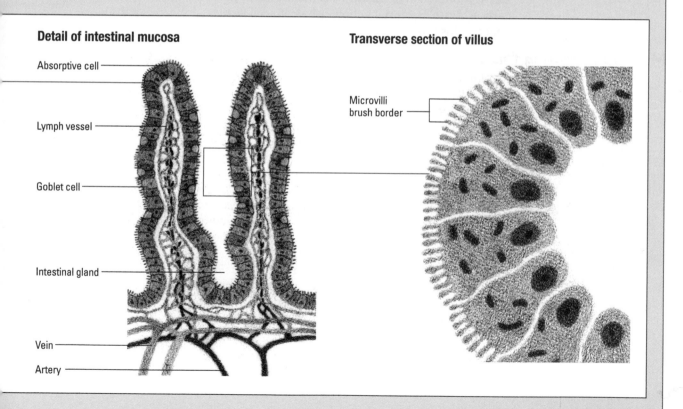

Detail of intestinal mucosa

Absorptive cell

Lymph vessel

Goblet cell

Intestinal gland

Vein

Artery

Transverse section of villus

Microvilli brush border

the exterior through two sphincters. The *internal sphincter* contains thick, circular smooth muscle under autonomic control; the *external sphincter* contains skeletal muscle under voluntary control.

Role in absorption

The large intestine produces no hormones or digestive enzymes; it continues the absorptive process. Through blood and lymph vessels in the submucosa, the proximal half of the large intestine absorbs all but about 100 ml of the remaining water in the colon. It also absorbs large amounts of both sodium and chloride.

Bacterial action

The large intestine harbors the bacteria *Escherichia coli*, *Enterobacter aerogenes*, *Clostridium perfringens*, and *Lactobacillus bifidus*. All of these bacteria help synthesize vitamin K and break down cellulose into a usable carbohydrate. Bacterial action also produces *flatus*, which helps propel stool toward the rectum.

Mucosa preparing for...

In addition, the mucosa of the large intestine produces *alkaline secretions* from tubular glands composed of goblet cells. This alkaline mucus lubricates the intestinal walls as food pushes through, protecting the mucosa from acidic bacterial action.

We're not all bad. Some of us bacteria aid GI function.

...mass movement

In the lower colon, long and relatively sluggish contractions cause propulsive waves, or *mass movements*. Normally occurring several times per day, these movements propel intestinal contents into the rectum and produce the urge to defecate.

Defecation normally results from the *defecation reflex*, a sensory and parasympathetic nerve-mediated response, along with the voluntary relaxation of the external anal sphincter. (See *GI changes with aging*.)

Senior moment

GI changes with aging

The physiologic changes that accompany aging usually prove less debilitating in the GI system than in most other body systems. Normal changes include diminished mucosal elasticity and reduced GI secretions which, in turn, modify some processes—for example, digestion and absorption. GI tract motility, bowel wall and anal sphincter tone, and abdominal muscle strength also may decrease with age. Any of these changes may cause complaints in an older patient, ranging from loss of appetite to constipation.

Changes in the oral cavity also occur. Tooth enamel wears away, leaving the teeth prone to cavities. Periodontal disease increases and the number of taste buds declines. The sense of smell diminishes and salivary gland secretion decreases, leading to appetite loss.

Liver changes

Normal physiologic changes in the liver include decreased liver weight, reduced regenerative capacity, and decreased blood flow to the liver. Because hepatic enzymes involved in oxidation and reduction markedly decline with age, the liver metabolizes drugs and detoxifies substances less efficiently.

Quick quiz

1. Which component of the GI system completes food digestion?

    A. Stomach
    B. Gallbladder
    C. Small intestine
    D. Large intestine

Answer: C. The small intestine completes the process of digestion.

2. One of the functions of the liver is:

    A. regulating gastrin secretion.
    B. storing vitamins A, C, and E.
    C. storing vitamins K, D, and B_{12}.
    D. detoxifying endogenous and exogenous toxins in plasma.

Answer: D. Among many other functions, the liver is responsible for detoxifying various exogenous and endogenous toxins in plasma.

3. Which GI hormone stimulates gastric secretion and motility?
- A. Gastrin
- B. Gastric inhibitory peptides
- C. Secretin
- D. Cholecystokinin

Answer: A. Gastrin is produced in the pyloric antrum and duodenal end mucosa and stimulates gastric secretion and motility.

4. In which phase of digestion does the stomach secrete the digestive juices hydrochloric acid and pepsin?
- A. Cephalic
- B. Gastric
- C. Intestinal
- D. Stomach emptying

Answer: A. By the time food is traveling toward the stomach, the cephalic phase — during which the stomach secretes digestive juices — has begun.

Scoring

☆☆☆ If you answered all four questions correctly, bravo! You've passed through the GI system with the greatest of ease!

☆☆ If you answered three questions correctly, super! You've chewed the fat of this system and it's time to move on.

☆ If you answered fewer than three questions correctly, don't worry! It might take a little longer to digest this material, but keep at it!

Nutrition and metabolism

Just the facts

In this chapter, you'll learn:

♦ roles of carbohydrates, proteins, and lipids in nutrition

♦ functions of vitamins and minerals in the body

♦ the way in which glucose is turned into energy

♦ role of hormones in metabolism.

Nutrition

Nutrition refers to the intake, assimilation, and utilization of nutrients. The crucial nutrients in foods must be broken down into components. Within cells, the products of digestion undergo further chemical reactions.

Metabolism refers to the sum of these chemical reactions. Through metabolism, food substances are transformed into energy or materials that the body can use or store.

Metabolism involves two processes:

☞ *anabolism* — synthesis of simple substances into complex ones

✌ *catabolism* — breakdown of complex substances into simpler ones or into energy.

Food
+
Metabolism =

Energy

Needed for nutrition

The body needs a continual supply of water and various nutrients for growth and repair. Virtually all nutrients come from digested food. The three major types of nutrients required by the body are carbohydrates, proteins, and lipids.

Needed for metabolism

Vitamins are essential for normal metabolism. They contribute to the enzyme reactions that promote the metabolism of carbohydrates, proteins, and lipids. *Minerals* are also important. They participate in such essential functions as enzyme metabolism and membrane transfer of essential elements. (See *The Food Guide Pyramid*.)

Carbohydrates

Carbohydrates are organic compounds composed of carbon, hydrogen, and oxygen; they yield 4 kcal/g when used for energy. Carbohydrates are classified as *monosaccha-*

> The energy in nutrients is measured in kilocalories — commonly just called calories. Adults need between 1,600 and 2,800 kcal daily, depending on their age, height, weight, and physical activity.

The Food Guide Pyramid

The Food Guide Pyramid suggests eating a large variety of foods (with emphasis on fruits, vegetables, and whole grain starches) for good health. In this diet, most of the fat comes from the milk and cheese and the meat, poultry, and eggs groups. Caloric intake ranges from 1,600 calories to 2,800 calories daily.

Fats, Oils, and Sweets Group
Use Sparingly

Milk, Yogurt, and Cheese Group
2 to 3 Servings

Meat, Poultry, Fish, Dry Beans, Eggs, and Nuts Group
2 to 3 Servings

Vegetable Group
3 to 5 Servings

Fruit Group
2 to 4 Servings

Bread, Cereal, Rice, and Pasta Group
6 to 11 Servings

Key: ● Fat (naturally occurring and added) ▲ Sugars (added)

Source: U.S. Department of Agriculture and U.S. Department of Health and Human Services.

rides, *disaccharides*, and *polysaccharides*. Sugars are carbohydrates and function as the body's primary energy source.

Monosaccharides

Monosaccharides are simple sugars that can't be split into smaller units by hydrolysis. They're subdivided into polyhydroxy aldehydes or ketones, based on whether the molecule consists of an aldehyde group or a ketone group.

The OH link

An aldehyde contains the characteristic group CHO. The term *polyhydroxy* refers to the linking of carbon atoms to an hydroxyl (OH) group.

CO is the key to ketone

A *ketone*, on the other hand, contains the carbonyl group CO and carbon groups attached to the carbonyl carbon.

Disaccharides

Disaccharides are synthesized from monosaccharides. A disaccharide molecule consists of two monosaccharides minus a water molecule. Examples of disaccharides include:
• *sucrose*, common table sugar, which is also found in some fruits and vegetables—a combination of a glucose molecule and a fructose molecule.
• *lactose*, the sugar found in milk—a combination of a glucose molecule and a galactose molecule.
• *maltose*, a sugar used in brewing and distilling—a combination of two glucose molecules.

Polysaccharides

Like disaccharides, *polysaccharides* are synthesized from monosaccharides. A polysaccharide consists of a long chain (*polymer*) of more than 10 monosaccharides linked by glycoside bonds. Polysaccharides are ingested and broken down into simple sugars and then used for fuel. Glycogen is an example of a polysaccharide. The body builds glycogen by using excess sugar (monosaccharides) and stores it for future use. When glycogen reserves are full, the liver converts the excess to fat.

Fiber is another example of a polysaccharide, but it can't be broken down into simple sugars. Thus, the body can't derive energy (fuel) from fiber.

Proteins

Proteins are complex nitrogenous organic compounds containing amino acid chains; some also contain sulfur and phosphorus. Proteins are used mainly for growth and repair of body tissues; when used for energy, they yield 4 kcal/g. Some proteins combine with lipids to form *lipoproteins* or with carbohydrates to form *glyco-proteins*.

The body uses proteins for growth and repair.

Amino acids

Amino acids are the building blocks of proteins. Each amino acid contains a carbon atom to which a carboxyl (COOH) group and an amino group are attached.

The bonds that link...

Amino acids unite by condensation of the COOH group on one amino acid with the amino group of the adjacent amino acid. This reaction releases a water molecule and creates a linkage called a *peptide bond*.

...and the acids that attract

The sequence and types of amino acids in the chain determine the nature of the protein. Each protein is synthesized on a ribosome as a straight chain. Chemical attractions between the amino acids in various parts of the chain cause the chain to coil or twist into a specific shape. A protein's shape, in turn, determines its function.

Lipids

Lipids are organic compounds that don't dissolve in water but do dissolve in alcohol and other organic solvents. Lipids are a concentrated form of fuel and yield approximately 9 kcal/g when used for energy. The major lipids include fats (the most common lipids), phospholipids, and steroids.

Memory jogger

Remember the three P's of proteins:

Peptide = 2 to 10 amino acids

Polypeptide = 10 or more amino acids

Protein = 50 or more amino acids.

Fats

A fat, or *triglyceride*, contains three molecules of fatty acid combined with one molecule of glycerol. A fatty acid is composed of a chain of carbon atoms with hydrogen and a few oxygen atoms attached. Fatty acid chains vary in length. Long-chain fatty acids (12 or more carbon atoms) are found in most food fats.

The glycerol example

Glycerol, for example, is a three-carbon compound (alcohol) with an OH group attached to each carbon atom. The COOH group on each fatty acid molecule joins to one OH group on the glycerol molecule; this results in the release of a water molecule. Linking of the COOH and OH groups produces an ester linkage.

Phospholipids

Phospholipids are complex lipids that are similar to fat but have a phosphorus- and nitrogen-containing compound that replaces one of the fatty acid molecules. Phospholipids are major structural components of cell membranes.

Steroids

Steroids are complex molecules in which the carbon atoms form four cyclic structures attached to various side chains. They contain no glycerol or fatty acid molecules. Examples of steroids include cholesterol, bile salts, and sex hormones.

Vitamins and minerals

Vitamins are organic compounds that are needed in small quantities for normal metabolism, growth, and development. Vitamins are classified as *water-soluble* or *fat-soluble*. Water-soluble vitamins include the B complex and C vitamins; fat-soluble vitamins include vitamins A, D, E, and K. (See *Guide to vitamins and minerals*, pages 220 to 222.)

Eat up! The body can't manufacture enough of us on its own

(Text continues on page 222.)

Guide to vitamins and minerals

Good health requires intake of adequate amounts of vitamins and minerals to meet the body's metabolic needs. A vitamin or mineral excess or deficiency can lead to various disorders. The chart below reviews major functions of vitamins and minerals and their food sources.

Vitamin or mineral	Major functions	Food sources
Water-soluble vitamins		
Vitamin C (ascorbic acid)	• Collagen production, fine bone and tooth formation, iodine conservation, healing, red blood cell (RBC) formation, infection resistance	• Fresh fruits and vegetables
Vitamin B_1 (thiamine)	• Blood formation, carbohydrate metabolism, circulation, digestion, growth, learning ability, muscle tone maintenance, central nervous system (CNS) maintenance	• Meats, fish, poultry, pork, molasses, brewer's yeast, brown rice, nuts, wheat germ, whole and enriched grains
Vitamin B_2 (riboflavin)	• RBC formation; energy metabolism; cell respiration; epithelial, eye, and mucosal tissue maintenance	• Meats, fish, poultry, milk, molasses, brewer's yeast, eggs, fruit, green leafy vegetables, nuts, whole grains
Vitamin B_6 (pyridoxine)	• Antibody formation, digestion, deoxyribonucleic acid (DNA) and ribonucleic acid (RNA) synthesis, fat and protein utilization, amino acid metabolism, hemoglobin production, CNS maintenance	• Meats, poultry, bananas, molasses, brewer's yeast, desiccated liver, fish, green leafy vegetables, peanuts, raisins, walnuts, wheat germ, whole grains
Folic acid (folacin, pteroylglutamic acid)	• Cell growth and reproduction, digestion, liver function, DNA and RNA formation, protein metabolism, RBC formation	• Citrus fruits, eggs, green leafy vegetables, milk products, organ meats, seafood, whole grains
Niacin (nicotinic acid, nicotinamide, niacinamide)	• Circulation, cholesterol level reduction, growth, hydrochloric acid production, metabolism (carbohydrate, protein, fat), sex hormone production	• Eggs, lean meats, milk products, organ meats, peanuts, poultry, seafood, whole grains
Vitamin B_{12} (cyanocobalamin)	• RBC formation, cellular and nutrient metabolism, tissue growth, nerve cell maintenance, appetite stimulation	• Beef, eggs, fish, milk products, organ meats, pork

Guide to vitamins and minerals (continued)

Vitamin or mineral	Major functions	Food sources
Fat-soluble vitamins		
Vitamin A	• Body tissue repair and maintenance, infection resistance, bone growth, nervous system development, cell membrane metabolism and structure, night vision	• Meat, milk, eggs, butter • Leafy green and yellow vegetables, yellow fruits (sources of carotene—a precursor to vitamin A)
Vitamin D (calciferol)	• Calcium and phosphorus metabolism (bone formation), myocardial function, nervous system maintenance, normal blood clotting	• Egg yolks, organ meats, butter, cod liver oil, fatty fish
Vitamin E (tocopherol)	• Aging retardation, anticlotting factor, diuresis, fertility, lung protection (antipollution), male potency, muscle and nerve cell membrane maintenance, myocardial perfusion, serum cholesterol reduction	• Butter, dark green vegetables, eggs, fruits, nuts, organ meats, vegetable oils, wheat germ
Vitamin K (menadione)	• Liver synthesis of prothrombin and other blood-clotting factors	• Green leafy vegetables, safflower oil, yogurt, liver, molasses • Also manufactured by bacteria that line the GI tract
Minerals		
Calcium	• Blood clotting, bone and tooth formation, cardiac rhythm, cell membrane permeability, muscle growth and contraction, nerve impulse transmission	• Cheese, milk, molasses, yogurt, whole grains, nuts, legumes, leafy vegetables
Chloride	• Maintenance of fluid, electrolyte, acid-base, and osmotic pressure balance	• Fruits, vegetables, table salt
Magnesium	• Acid-base balance, metabolism, protein synthesis, muscle relaxation, cellular respiration, nerve impulse transmission	• Green leafy vegetables, nuts, seafood, cocoa, whole grains
Phosphorus	• Bone and tooth formation, cell growth and repair, energy production	• Eggs, fish, grains, meats, poultry, milk, milk products

(continued)

Guide to vitamins and minerals *(continued)*

Vitamin or mineral	Major functions	Food source
Minerals *(continued)*		
Potassium	• Heartbeat, muscle contraction, nerve impulse transmission, rapid growth, fluid distribution and osmotic pressure balance, acid-base balance	• Seafood, molasses, vegetables, fruits, nuts
Sodium	• Cellular fluid level maintenance, muscle contraction, acid-base balance, cell permeability, muscle function, nerve impulse transmission	• Cheese, milk, salt, processed foods, canned soups, fast food, soy sauce
Fluoride (fluorine)	• Bone and tooth formation	• Drinking water, seafood
Iodine	• Thyroid hormone production, energy production, metabolism, physical and mental development	• Kelp, salt (iodized), seafood
Iron	• Growth (in children), hemoglobin production, stress and disease resistance, cellular respiration, oxygen transport	• Egg yolks, meats, poultry, wheat germ, liver, oysters, enriched breads and cereals, green vegetables, molasses
Selenium	• Immune mechanisms, mitochondrial adenosine triphosphate synthesis, cellular protection	• Seafood, meats, liver, eggs
Zinc	• Burn and wound healing, carbohydrate digestion, metabolism (carbohydrate, fat, protein), prostate gland function, reproductive organ growth and development, cell growth	• Liver, mushrooms, seafood, soybeans, spinach, meats

Minerals

Minerals are inorganic substances that play important roles in:
• enzyme metabolism
• membrane transfer of essential compounds
• regulation of acid-base balance
• osmotic pressure
• muscle contractility
• nerve impulse transmission
• growth.

Minerals are found in bones, hemoglobin, thyroxine, teeth, and organs. They're classified as *major minerals* (more than 0.005% of body weight) or *trace minerals* (less than 0.005% of body weight). Major minerals include calcium, chloride, magnesium, phosphorus, potassium, and sodium. Trace minerals include chromium, cobalt, copper, fluorine, iodine, iron, manganese, molybdenum, selenium, and zinc.

> Gotta split! During hydrolysis, a compound unites with water and then splits into simpler compounds.

Absorption and digestion

Nutrients must be digested in the GI tract by enzymes that split large units into smaller ones. In this process, called *hydrolysis*, a compound unites with water and then splits into simpler compounds. The smaller units are then absorbed from the small intestine and transported to the liver through the portal venous system.

Carbohydrate digestion and absorption

Enzymes break down complex carbohydrates. In the oral cavity, *salivary amylase* initiates starch hydrolysis into disaccharides. In the small intestine, *pancreatic amylase* continues this process.

Splitting, hydrolyzing...

Disaccharide enzymes in the intestinal mucosa hydrolyze disaccharides into monosaccharides. Lactase splits the compound lactose into glucose and galactose, and sucrase hydrolyzes the compound sucrose into glucose and fructose.

... and movin' along

Monosaccharides, such as glucose, fructose, and galactose, are absorbed through the intestinal mucosa and are then transported through the portal venous system to the liver. There, enzymes convert fructose and galactose to glucose.

Ribonucleases and deoxyribonucleases break down nucleotides from deoxyribonucleic acid and ribonucleic acid into pentoses and nitrogen-containing compounds (nitrogen bases). Like glucose, these compounds are absorbed through the intestinal mucosa.

Protein digestion and absorption

Enzymes digest proteins by hydrolyzing the peptide bonds that link the amino acids of the protein chains. This process of hydrolyzation restores water molecules.

Gastric pepsin breaks proteins into:

- polypeptides
- pancreatic trypsin
- chymotrypsin
- carboxypeptidase, which converts polypeptides to peptides.

The breakdown lane

Intestinal mucosal peptidases break down peptides into their constituent amino acids. After being absorbed through the intestinal mucosa by active transport mechanisms, these amino acids travel through the portal venous system to the liver. The liver converts the amino acids not needed for protein synthesis into glucose.

Amino acids: Enter here and prepare to convert.

Lipid digestion and absorption

Most fat digestion occurs in the small intestine. Pancreatic lipase breaks down fats and phospholipids into a mixture of glycerol, short- and long-chain fatty acids, and monoglycerides. The portal venous system then carries these substances to the liver. Lipase hydrolyzes the bonds between glycerol and fatty acids — a process that restores the water molecules released when the bonds were formed.

On a short leash...

Glycerol diffuses directly through the mucosa. Short-chain fatty acids diffuse into the intestinal epithelial cells and are carried to the liver via the portal venous system.

...or on a long one

Long-chain fatty acids and monoglycerides in the intestine dissolve in the bile salt micelles and then diffuse into the intestinal epithelial cells. There, lipase breaks down absorbed monoglycerides into glycerol and fatty acids. In the smooth endoplasmic reticulum of the epithelial cells, fatty acids and glycerol recombine to form fats.

Chylomicrons

Along with a small amount of cholesterol and phospholipid, triglycerides are coated with a thin layer of protein to form lipoprotein particles called *chylomicrons*. Chylomicrons collect in the intestinal lacteals (lymphatic vessels) and are carried through lymphatic channels. After entering the circulation through the thoracic duct, they're distributed to body cells.

Stored away for later

In the cells, fats are extracted from the chylomicrons and broken down by enzymes into fatty acids and glycerol. Then they're absorbed and recombined in fat cells, reforming triglycerides for storage and later use.

Carbohydrate metabolism

Carbohydrates are the preferred energy fuel of human cells. Most of the carbohydrates in absorbed food is quickly catabolized for the release of energy.

Glucose to energy

All ingested carbohydrates are converted to glucose, the body's main energy source. Glucose not needed for immediate energy is stored as glycogen or converted to lipids.

Energy from glucose catabolism is generated in three phases:

☝ glycolysis

✌ Krebs cycle (also called the citric acid cycle)

🤟 the electron transport system. (See *Tracking the glucose pathway*, page 226.)

Glycolysis, which occurs in the cell cytoplasm, doesn't use oxygen. The other two phases, which occur in mitochondria, do use oxygen.

This whole nutrition and metabolism thing is pretty simple; it's about getting energy to do things!

Now I get it!

Tracking the glucose pathway

Glucose catabolism generates energy in three phases: glycolysis, Krebs cycle, and the electron transport system The flowchart below summarizes the first two phases.

Glycolysis
Glycolysis, the first phase, breaks apart one molecule of glucose to form two molecules of pyruvate, which yields energy in the form of adenosine triphosphate and acetyl coenzyme A (CoA).

Krebs cycle
The second phase, the Krebs cycle, continues carbohydrate metabolism. Fragments of acetyl CoA join to oxaloacetic acid to form citric acid. The CoA molecule breaks off from the acetyl group and may form more acetyl CoA molecules. Citric acid is first converted into intermediate compounds and then back into oxaloacetic acid. The Krebs cycle also liberates carbon dioxide.

Electron transport system
In the third phase of glucose catabolism, molecules on the inner mitochondrial membrane attract electrons from hydrogen atoms and carry them through oxidation-reduction reactions in the mitochondria. The hydrogen ions produced in the Krebs cycle then combine with oxygen to form water.

Glucose is the body's main energy source.

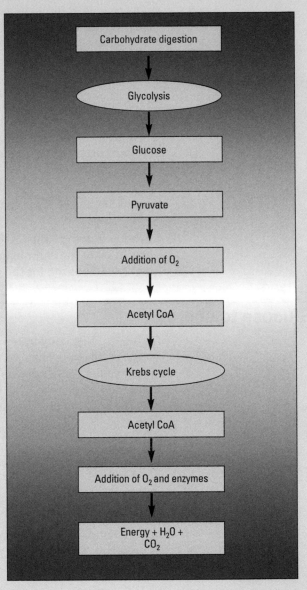

Carbohydrate digestion

Glycolysis

Glucose

Pyruvate

Addition of O_2

Acetyl CoA

Krebs cycle

Acetyl CoA

Addition of O_2 and enzymes

Energy + H_2O + CO_2

Glycolysis

Glycolysis refers to the process by which enzymes break down the 6-carbon glucose molecule into two 3-carbon molecules of pyruvic acid (pyruvate). Glycolysis yields energy in the form of adenosine triphosphate (ATP).

Cruising the glucose pathway

Next, pyruvic acid releases a carbon dioxide (CO_2) molecule and is converted in the mitochondria to a two-carbon acetyl fragment, which combines with a complex organic compound called *coenzyme A (CoA)* to form acetyl CoA.

Krebs cycle

The second phase in glucose catabolism is the Krebs cycle. It's the pathway by which a molecule of acetyl CoA is oxidized by enzymes to yield energy.

Carbons, carbons everywhere

The two-carbon acetyl fragments of acetyl CoA enter the Krebs cycle by joining to the four-carbon compound oxaloacetic acid to form citric acid, a six-carbon compound. In this process, the CoA molecule detaches from the acetyl group, becoming available to form more acetyl CoA molecules. Enzymes convert citric acid into intermediate compounds and eventually convert it back into oxaloacetic acid. Then the cycle can begin again.

In addition to liberating CO_2 and generating energy, each turn of the Krebs cycle releases hydrogen atoms, which are picked up by the coenzymes nicotinamide adenine dinucleotide (NAD) and flavin adenine dinucleotide (FAD).

> The last step of carbohydrate catabolism is electron transport.

Electron transport system

The electron transport system is the last phase of carbohydrate catabolism. In this phase, carrier molecules on the inner mitochondrial membrane pick up electrons from the hydrogen atoms carried by NAD and FAD. (Each hydrogen atom contains a hydrogen ion and an electron.) These carrier molecules transport the electrons through a series of enzyme-catalyzed oxidation-reduction reactions in the mitochondria.

Oxygen attraction

Oxygen plays a crucial role by attracting electrons along the chain of carriers in the transport system. During oxidation, a chemical compound loses electrons; during reduction, it gains electrons. These reactions release the energy contained in the electrons and generate ATP.

After passing through the electron transport system, the hydrogen ions produced in the Krebs cycle combine with oxygen to form water.

> I convert glucose into glycogen or lipids.

Liver and muscle cells

Both the liver and muscle cells help to regulate blood glucose levels.

Liver

When glucose levels exceed the body's immediate needs, hormones stimulate the liver to convert glucose into glycogen or lipids. Glycogen forms through glycogenesis; lipids form through lipogenesis.

Glucose shortage

When the blood glucose level drops excessively, the liver can form glucose by two processes:
• breakdown of glycogen to glucose through glycogenolysis
• synthesis of glucose from amino acids through gluconeogenesis.

> Look out glycogen! I'm breaking you down and creating energy!

Muscle cells

Muscle cells can convert glucose to glycogen for storage. However, they lack the enzymes to convert glycogen back to glucose when needed. During vigorous muscular activity, when oxygen requirements exceed the oxygen supply, muscle cells break down glycogen to yield lactic acid and energy. Lactic acid then builds up in the muscles, and muscle glycogen is depleted.

Glycogen returns

Some of the lactic acid diffuses from muscle cells, is transported to the liver, and is reconverted to glycogen. The liver converts the newly formed glycogen to glucose, which travels through the bloodstream to the muscles and reforms into glycogen.

Energize!

When muscle exertion stops, some of the accumulated lactic acid converts back to pyruvic acid. Pyruvic acid is oxidized completely to yield energy by means of Krebs cycle and the electron transport system.

Protein metabolism

Proteins are absorbed as amino acids and carried by the portal venous system to the liver, and then throughout the body by blood. Absorbed amino acids mix with other amino acids in the body's amino acid pool. These other amino acids may be synthesized by the body from other substances such as *keto acids*, or they may be produced by protein breakdown.

Amino acid conversion

The body can't store amino acids; instead, it converts them to protein or glucose or catabolizes them to provide energy. Before these changes can occur, however, amino acids must be transformed by deamination or transamination.

Deamination

In *deamination*, an amino group ($-NH_2$) splits off from an amino acid molecule to form one molecule of ammonia and one of keto acid. Most of the ammonia is converted to urea and excreted in the urine.

Transamination

In *transamination*, an amino group is exchanged for a keto group in a keto acid through the action of transaminase enzymes. During this process, the amino acid is converted to a keto acid and the original keto acid is converted to an amino acid.

Amino acid synthesis

Proteins are synthesized from 20 amino acids from the body's amino acid pool. (See *Essential and nonessential amino acids*.)

Power station

Amino acids not used for protein synthesis can be converted to keto acids and metabolized by the Krebs cycle and the electron transport system to produce energy.

Fat chance

Amino acids can also be converted to other nutrients such as fats. Those amino acids not used for protein synthesis may be converted to pyruvic acid and then to acetyl CoA. The acetyl CoA fragments condense to form long-chain fatty acids — a process that is the reverse of fatty acid breakdown. These fatty acids then combine with glycerol to form fats.

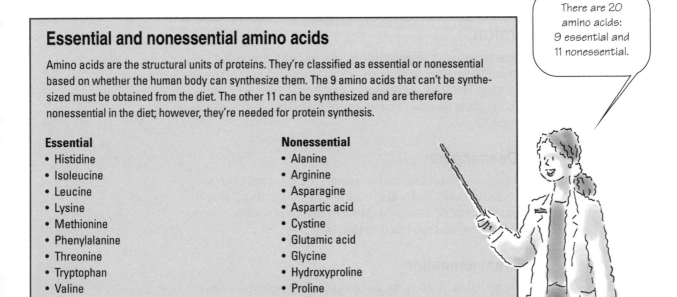

Essential and nonessential amino acids

Amino acids are the structural units of proteins. They're classified as essential or nonessential based on whether the human body can synthesize them. The 9 amino acids that can't be synthesized must be obtained from the diet. The other 11 can be synthesized and are therefore nonessential in the diet; however, they're needed for protein synthesis.

Essential
- Histidine
- Isoleucine
- Leucine
- Lysine
- Methionine
- Phenylalanine
- Threonine
- Tryptophan
- Valine

Nonessential
- Alanine
- Arginine
- Asparagine
- Aspartic acid
- Cystine
- Glutamic acid
- Glycine
- Hydroxyproline
- Proline
- Serine
- Tyrosine

There are 20 amino acids: 9 essential and 11 nonessential.

Going glucose

Amino acids can also be converted to glucose. They're first converted to pyruvic acid, which may then be converted to glucose.

Lipid metabolism

Lipids are stored in adipose tissue within cells until they're required for use as fuel. When needed for energy, each fat molecule is hydrolyzed to glycerol and three molecules of fatty acids. Glycerol can be converted to pyruvic acid and then to acetyl CoA, which enters the Krebs cycle.

Ketone body formation

The liver normally forms ketone bodies from acetyl CoA fragments, derived largely from fatty acid catabolism. Acetyl CoA molecules yield three types of ketone bodies: acetoacetic acid, beta-hydroxybutyric acid, and acetone.

Acetoacetic acid results from the combination of two acetyl CoA molecules and the subsequent release of CoA from these molecules.

Beta-hydroxybutyric acid forms when hydrogen is added to the oxygen atom in the acetoacetic acid molecule. The term *beta* indicates the location of the carbon atom containing the OH group.

Acetone forms when the COOH group of acetoacetic acid releases CO_2. Muscle tissue, brain tissue, and other tissues oxidize these ketone bodies for energy.

> Along with other tissues, I oxidize ketone bodies for energy.

Excessive ketone formation

Under certain conditions, the body produces more ketone bodies than it can oxidize for energy. Such conditions include fasting, starvation, and uncontrolled diabetes (in which the body can't break down glucose). The body must then use fat, rather than glucose, as its primary energy source.

Ketone cops

Use of fat instead of glucose for energy leads to an excess of ketone bodies. This condition disturbs the body's

Senior moment

Nutrition-related changes with aging

As a person ages, caloric needs decrease. Protein, vitamin, and mineral requirements usually remain the same throughout life. The body's ability to process these nutrients, however, is also affected by the aging process.

Physiologic changes

Diminished intestinal motility typically accompanies aging and may cause GI disorders such as constipation. Physical inactivity, emotional stress, medications, and nutritionally inadequate diets of soft, refined foods that are low in dietary fiber can also cause constipation. Laxative abuse results in the rapid transport of food through the GI tract, decreasing digestion and absorption. Fecal incontinence may also occur in elderly patients.

Other physiologic changes that can affect nutrition in an older patient include:
• decreased renal function, causing greater susceptibility to dehydration and formation of renal calculi
• loss of calcium and nitrogen (in people who aren't ambulatory)
• diminished enzyme activity and gastric secretions

• reduced pepsin and hydrochloric acid secretion, which tends to diminish the absorption of calcium and vitamins B_1 and B_2
• decreased salivary flow and diminished sense of taste, which may reduce the appetite and increase a person's consumption of sweet and spicy foods
• diminished intestinal motility and peristalsis of the large intestine
• thinning of tooth enamel, causing teeth to become more brittle
• decreased biting force
• diminished gag reflex.

Affecting factors

Nutritional status can be affected by such socioeconomic and psychological factors as loneliness, decline of the older person's importance in the family, susceptibility to nutritional quackery, and lack of money or transportation, which limit access to nutritious foods. In addition, some conditions that are common among older people can affect mobility and, therefore, the ability to obtain or prepare food or feed oneself.

normal acid-base balance and homeostatic mechanisms, leading to ketosis.

Lipid formation

Excess amino acids can be converted to fat through keto acid–acetyl CoA conversion. Glucose may be converted to pyruvic acid and then to acetyl CoA, which is converted into fatty acids and then fat (in much the same way that amino acids are converted into fat). (See *Nutrition-related changes with aging*.)

Hormonal regulation of metabolism

Normal body functions necessitate that blood glucose levels stay within a certain range.

Now I get it!

How insulin affects blood glucose level

Unlike most hormones, insulin tends to decrease the blood glucose level. It does this by helping glucose to enter cells, thereby promoting glycogenesis and stimulating glucose catabolism.

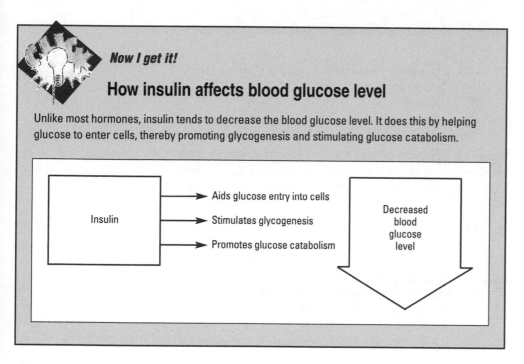

Insulin → Aids glucose entry into cells

→ Stimulates glycogenesis

→ Promotes glucose catabolism

Decreased blood glucose level

Glucose going up...

Hormones regulate the blood glucose level by stimulating the metabolic processes that restore a normal level in response to blood glucose changes. (See *How insulin affects blood glucose level.*)

...and going down!

Insulin, produced by the pancreatic islet cells, is the only hormone that significantly reduces the blood glucose level. In addition to promoting cell uptake and use of glucose as an energy source, insulin promotes glucose storage as glycogen (glycogenesis) and lipids (lipogenesis).

Quick quiz

1. Which type of nutrient yields 9 kcal/g when used for energy?
- A. Proteins
- B. Carbohydrates
- C. Lipids
- D. Vitamins

Answer: C. Lipids are a concentrated form of fuel and yield 9 kcal/g.

2. Which hormone decreases the blood glucose level?
  A. Epinephrine
  B. Cortisol
  C. Insulin
  D. Glycogen

Answer: C. Insulin is the only hormone that significantly reduces blood glucose. It does so by aiding glucose entry into cells, thereby stimulating glycogenesis and promoting glucose catabolism.

3. Essential amino acids are:
  A. organic compounds that are needed in small amounts for normal metabolism, growth, and development.
  B. organic compounds that don't dissolve in water but do dissolve in alcohol and other organic solvents.
  C. the structural unit of protein that doesn't need to be obtained from the diet.
  D. the structural unit of protein that must be obtained from the diet.

Answer: D. Essential amino acids can't be synthesized in the body and, therefore, must be obtained from the diet.

4. Which vitamin is involved in prothrombin synthesis and other blood-clotting factors?
  A. Vitamin K
  B. Vitamin E
  C. Vitamin B_{12}
  D. Vitamin B_6

Answer: A. Vitamin K is involved in liver synthesis of prothrombin and other blood-clotting factors.

Scoring

☆☆☆ If you answered all four questions correctly, hooray! You've digested a healthy dose of dense clinical material.

☆☆ If you answered three questions correctly, remarkable! You'll soon be a master of metabolism.

☆ If you answered fewer than three questions correctly, get energized! You've got four more quick quizzes to go!

Urinary system

Just the facts

In this chapter, you'll learn:

♦ major structures of the urinary system

♦ functions of the kidneys, ureters, bladder, and urethra

♦ the way in which urine is formed

♦ role of hormones in the urinary system.

Structures of the urinary system

The urinary system consists of:
- two kidneys
- two ureters
- the bladder
- the urethra.

Working together, these structures remove wastes from the body, help to govern acid-base balance by retaining and excreting hydrogen ions, regulate fluid and electrolyte balance, and assist in blood pressure control.

Think of us as the body's plumbers. Together with the ureters, bladder, and urethra, we do everything from removing wastes...

...to balancing fluids and electrolytes, to keeping blood pressure in check.

Kidneys

The *kidneys* are bean-shaped, highly vascular organs. Each kidney consists of three regions:
- renal cortex (outer region)
- renal medulla (middle region)
- renal pelvis (inner region). (See *A close look at the kidneys.*)

Filtering station

The *renal cortex*, the outer region, contains blood-filtering mechanisms and is protected by a fibrous capsule and layers of fat.

Renal wonder

The *renal medulla*, the middle region of the kidney, contains 8 to 12 renal pyramids — striated wedges that are composed mostly of tubular structures. The tapered portion of each pyramid empties into a cuplike calyx. These calyces channel formed urine from the pyramids into the *renal pelvis*.

> ### My three regions
>
> - The *renal cortex* (outer region) contains about 1.25 million renal tubules.
>
> - The *renal medulla* (middle region) functions as my collecting chamber.
>
> - The *renal pelvis* (inner region) receives urine through the major calyces.

Keeping kidneys safe

The kidneys are protected in front by the contents of the abdomen and behind by the muscles attached to the vertebral column. A layer of fat surrounding each kidney offers further protection.

Adrenal influence

On top of each kidney lies an adrenal gland. These glands are affected by the release of renin from the kidneys and, in turn, affect the renal system by influencing blood pressure as well as sodium and water retention in the kidneys.

No shortage of blood

Each kidney is supplied with blood by a renal artery, which subdivides into several branches when it enters the kidney. The kidneys are highly vascular (meaning that they contain a lot of blood vessels), receiving about 20% of the blood pumped by the heart each minute.

All in a day's work

Together, these tissues allow the kidneys to perform their many functions, including:

Zoom in

A close look at the kidneys

The kidneys are located in the lumbar area, with the right kidney situated slightly lower than the left to make room for the liver, which is just above it. The position of the kidneys shifts somewhat with changes in body position. Covering the kidneys are the true or fibrous capsule, perirenal fat, and renal fasciae.

Blood's cleansing journey

The kidneys receive waste-filled blood from the renal artery, which branches off the abdominal aorta. After passing through a complicated network of smaller blood vessels and nephrons, the filtered blood returns to the circulation by way of the renal vein, which empties into the inferior vena cava.

Continuing the cleanup

The kidneys excrete waste products that the nephrons remove from the blood; these excretions combine with other waste fluids (such as urea, creatinine, phosphates, and sulfates) to form urine. An action called *peristalsis* (the circular contraction and relaxation of a tube-shaped structure) passes the urine through the ureters and into the urinary bladder. When the bladder has filled, nerves in the bladder wall relax the sphincter. In conjunction with a voluntary stimulus, this relaxation causes urine to pass into the urethra for elimination from the body.

- elimination of wastes and excess ions (in the form of urine)
- blood filtration (by regulating chemical composition and blood volume)
- maintenance of fluid-electrolyte and acid-base balances

• production and release of renin to promote angiotensin II activation and aldosterone production in the adrenal gland
• production of erythropoietin (a hormone that stimulates red blood cell [RBC] production) and enzymes (such as renin, which governs blood pressure and kidney function)
• conversion of vitamin D to a more active form.

The nephron

Within the kidney, the *nephron* serves as the basic structural and functional unit. (See *Structure of the nephron.*)

Filter, reabsorb, and secrete

The nephrons perform two main functions:
• mechanically filtrating fluids, wastes, electrolytes, acids, and bases into the tubular system
• selectively reabsorbing and secreting ions, allowing precise control of fluid and electrolyte balance.

Part and parcel

Each nephron consists of a tubular apparatus called the *glomerulus* as well as a collecting duct. The glomerulus is located inside a glomerular capsule, or *Bowman's capsule*, and consists of a cluster of capillaries.

Totally tubular

The nephron is divided into three portions. The portion nearest the glomerular capsule is the *proximal convoluted tubule.* The second portion, the *loop of Henle,* has an ascending and a descending limb. The third portion, the one farthest from the glomerular capsule, is the *distal convoluted tubule.* Its distal end joins the far ends of neighboring nephrons, forming a larger collecting tubule.

Positively loopy

The glomeruli and proximal and distal tubules of the nephron are located in the renal cortex. The long loops of Henle, together with their accompanying blood vessels and collecting tubules, form the renal pyramids in the medulla.

Water, water everywhere

The proximal convoluted tubules have freely permeable cell membranes. This allows reabsorption of nearly all the filtrate's glucose, amino acids, metabolites, and elec-

Zoom in

Structure of the nephron

The *nephron* is the kidney's basic functional unit and the site of urine formation. The renal artery, a large branch of the abdominal aorta, carries blood to each kidney. Blood flows through the interlobular artery (running between the lobes of the kidneys) to the afferent arteriole, which conveys blood to the glomerulus. Blood passes through the glomerulus into the efferent arteriole and into the peritubular capillaries, venules, and the interlobular vein. The peritubular capillary network of vessels then supplies blood to the tubules of the nephron.

Proximal convoluted tubule

Distal convoluted tubule

Collecting tubule

Peritubular capillaries

Bowman's capsule

Glomerulus

Afferent arteriole

Efferent arteriole

Interlobular artery and vein

Arcuate artery and vein

Ascending loop of Henle

Descending loop of Henle

trolytes into nearby capillaries as well as allowing for the circulation of large amounts of water.

Time to concentrate

By the time the filtrate enters the descending limb of the loop of Henle, its water content has been reduced by 70%.

Senior moment

Urinary changes with aging

As a person ages, changes in the kidneys and bladder can affect urinary system function.

Kidneys
After age 40, kidney function may diminish; if the person lives to age 90, it may decrease by as much as 50%. Age-related changes in kidney vasculature that disturb glomerular hemodynamics result in a decline in glomerular filtration rate. Reduced cardiac output and age-related atherosclerotic changes cause kidney blood flow to decrease by 53%. In addition, tubular reabsorption and renal concentrating ability decline because the size and number of functioning nephrons decrease.

Bladder
As a person ages, bladder muscles weaken. This may lead to incomplete bladder emptying and chronic urine retention—predisposing the bladder to infection.

And the rest
Other age-related changes that affect renal function include diminished kidney size, impaired renal clearance of drugs, reduced bladder size and capacity, and decreased renal ability to respond to variations in sodium intake. By age 70, blood urea nitrogen levels rise by 21%. Residual urine, frequency of urination, and nocturia also increase with age.

At this point, the filtrate contains a high concentration of salts, chiefly sodium. As the filtrate moves deeper into the medulla and the loop of Henle, osmosis draws even more water into the extracellular spaces, further concentrating the filtrate.

Readjust and exit

After the filtrate enters the ascending limb, its concentration is readjusted by the transport of ions into the tubule. This transport continues until the filtrate enters the distal convoluted tubule. (*See Urinary changes with aging.*)

Ureters

The *ureters* are fibromuscular tubes that connect each kidney to the bladder. Because the left kidney is higher than the right kidney, the left ureter is usually slightly longer than the right ureter.

Triple protection

Each ureter is surrounded by a three-layered wall. (See *Three layers of the ureter.*)

Three layers of the ureter

Each ureter has a three-layered wall:
• The *mucosa*, the innermost layer, contains the transitional epithelium.
• The *muscularis*, the middle layer, contains smooth muscle layers.
• Extensions of the *fibrous coat*, the outer layer, hold the ureter in place.

Riding the waves

The ureters act as conduits that carry urine from the kidneys to the bladder. Peristaltic waves occurring one to five times each minute channel urine along the ureters toward the bladder.

Bladder

The *bladder* is a hollow, sphere-shaped, muscular organ in the pelvis. It lies anterior and inferior to the pelvic cavity and posterior to the *symphysis pubis* (the joint between the two pubic bones). Its function is to store urine. In a normal adult, bladder capacity ranges from 500 to 600 ml. If the amount of stored urine exceeds bladder capacity, the bladder distends above the symphysis pubis.

Good things come in threes

The base of the bladder contains three openings that form a triangular area called the *trigone*. Two of the openings connect the bladder to the ureters, while the third connects the bladder to the urethra.

A matter of reflex

Urination results from involuntary (reflex) and voluntary (learned or intentional) processes. When urine fills the bladder, parasympathetic nerve fibers in the bladder wall cause the bladder to contract and the *internal sphincter* (located at the internal urethral orifice) to relax. The cerebrum, in a voluntary reaction, then causes the external sphincter to relax and urination to begin. This is called the *micturition* reflex.

Urination is the result of two processes — one voluntary and one involuntary.

Urethra

The *urethra* is a small duct that channels urine from the bladder to the outside of the body.

Female connections

In the female, the urethra is embedded in the anterior wall of the vagina behind the symphysis pubis. The urethra connects the bladder with an external opening, or *urethral meatus*, located anterior to the vaginal opening.

The female urethra is composed of an inner layer of mucous membrane, a middle layer of spongy tissue, and an outer layer of muscle.

Male extensions

In the male, the urethra passes vertically through the *prostate* gland and then extends through the urogenital diaphragm and penis. The male urethra serves as a passageway for semen as well as urine.

Urine formation

Urine formation is one of the main functions of the urinary system. Urine formation results from three processes that occur in the nephrons: glomerular filtration, tubular reabsorption, and tubular secretion. (See *How the kidneys form urine.*)

A mine of minerals

When formed, normal urine consists of water, sodium, chloride, potassium, calcium, magnesium, sulfates, phosphates, bicarbonates, uric acid, ammonium ions, creatinine, and *urobilinogen* (a derivative of bilirubin resulting from the action of intestinal bacteria). A few leukocytes and RBCs (and, in males, some spermatozoa) may enter the urine as it passes from the kidney to the ureteral orifice. When a person is taking drugs that are normally excreted in urine, the urine contains those substances as well.

Kidneys in charge

The kidneys can vary the amount of substances reabsorbed and secreted in the nephrons, changing the composition of excreted urine.

Controlling the flow

Total daily urine output averages 720 to 2,400 ml, varying with fluid intake and climate. For example, after drinking a large volume of fluid, a person's urine output increases as the body rapidly excretes excess water. If a person restricts or decreases water intake or ingests excessive amounts of sodium, urine output decreases as the body retains water to restore normal fluid concentration.

We'd better get busy! We process up to 300 glasses of water every day!

Now I get it!

How the kidneys form urine

Urine formation occurs in three steps: glomerular filtration, tubular reabsorption, and tubular secretion.

Step 1: Filter

As blood flows into the glomerulus, filtration occurs. Active transport from the proximal convoluted tubules leads to reabsorption of sodium (Na^+) and glucose into nearby circulation. *Osmosis* then causes water (H_2O) reabsorption.

Step 2: Reabsorb

In tubular reabsorption, a substance moves from the filtrate in the distal convoluted tubules to the peritubular capillaries. Active transport results in Na^+, potassium (K^+), and glucose reabsorption. The presence of antidiuretic hormone causes H_2O reabsorption.

Step 3: Secrete

In tubular secretion, a substance moves from the peritubular capillaries into the tubular filtrate. Peritubular capillaries then secrete ammonia (NH_3) and hydrogen (H^+) into the distal tubules via active transport.

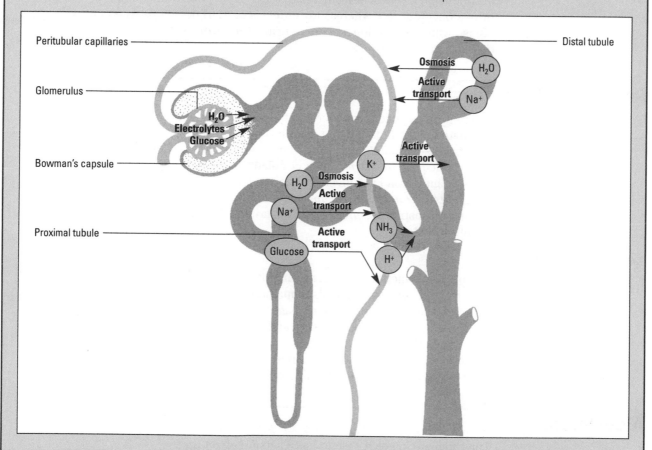

Hormones and the urinary system

Hormones play a major role in the urinary system, including helping the body to manage tubular reabsorption and secretion. Hormones affecting the urinary system include:

- antidiuretic hormone
- angiotensin I
- angiotensin II
- aldosterone
- erythropoietin.

Antidiuretic hormone

Antidiuretic hormone (ADH) regulates levels of urine output. High levels of ADH increase water absorption and urine concentration, whereas lower levels of ADH decrease water absorption and dilute urine. (See *How antidiuretic hormone works.*)

Renin-angiotensin system

Renin is an enzyme that's secreted by the kidneys and circulated in the blood. Renin itself has no effect on blood pressure, but it leads to the formation of the hormone called *angiotensin I.* As it circulates through the lungs, angiotensin I is converted into *angiotensin II* by *angiotensin-converting enzyme.* Angiotensin II exerts a powerful constricting effect on the arterioles. In this way, it can raise blood pressure.

The best defense

The primary function of the renin-angiotensin system is to serve as a defense mechanism, maintaining blood pressure in situations such as hemorrhage and extreme sodium depletion. Low blood pressure and low levels of sodium passing through the kidneys are two of the three factors that stimulate the kidneys to release renin. (The third is stimulation of the sympathetic nervous system.)

Aldosterone

The renin-angiotensin system has a second effect that makes it even more potent; it acts on the adrenal gland to

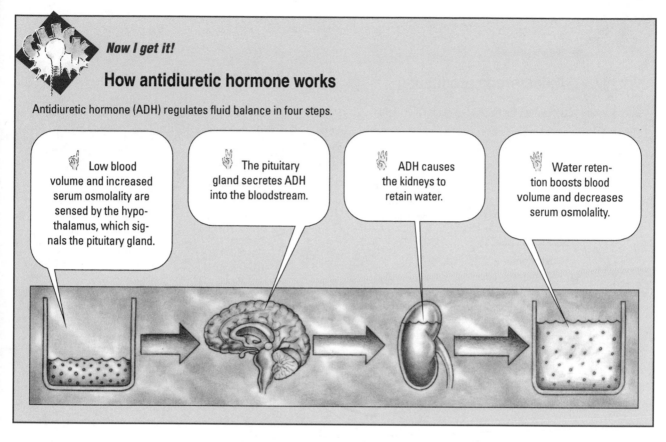

Now I get it!

How antidiuretic hormone works

Antidiuretic hormone (ADH) regulates fluid balance in four steps.

> ☝ Low blood volume and increased serum osmolality are sensed by the hypothalamus, which signals the pituitary gland.

> ✌ The pituitary gland secretes ADH into the bloodstream.

> 🖐 ADH causes the kidneys to retain water.

> ✌ Water retention boosts blood volume and decreases serum osmolality.

release *aldosterone*. (See *Aldosterone production*, page 246.)

BP assist

Aldosterone is produced by the adrenal cortex. It facilitates tubular reabsorption by regulating sodium retention and helping to control potassium secretion by epithelial cells in the tubules.

When serum potassium levels rise, the adrenal cortex responds by increasing aldosterone secretion. This, in turn, causes sodium retention, thereby raising blood pressure. (See *How aldosterone works*, page 247.)

Erythropoietin

The kidneys secrete the hormone *erythropoietin* in response to low arterial oxygen tension. The hormone trav-

Now I get it!

Aldosterone production

Aldosterone (a hormone that helps to regulate fluid balance) is released by the adrenal gland through the actions of the renin-angiotensin system.

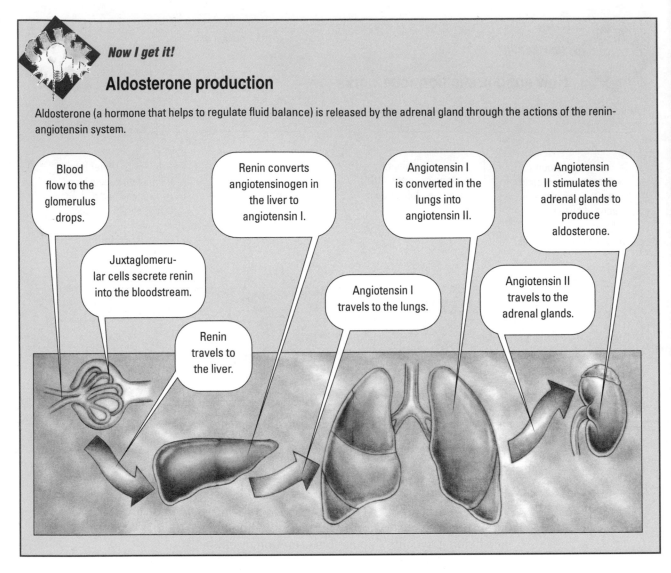

Blood flow to the glomerulus drops.

Juxtaglomeru-lar cells secrete renin into the bloodstream.

Renin travels to the liver.

Renin converts angiotensinogen in the liver to angiotensin I.

Angiotensin I travels to the lungs.

Angiotensin I is converted in the lungs into angiotensin II.

Angiotensin II travels to the adrenal glands.

Angiotensin II stimulates the adrenal glands to produce aldosterone.

els to the bone marrow, where it stimulates increased RBC production.

A balancing act

The kidneys also regulate calcium and phosphorus balance by filtering and reabsorbing approximately half of unbound serum calcium. In addition, the kidneys activate vitamin D_3, a compound that promotes intestinal calcium absorption and regulates phosphate excretion.

(Text continues on page 247.)

Incredibly Easy miniguide to physiology: The reflex arc

The reflex arc—a neural relay cycle for quick motor response to a harmful sensory stimulus—requires a sensory (afferent) neuron and a motor (efferent) neuron. The stimulus triggers a sensory impulse, which travels along the dorsal root to the spinal cord. There, two synaptic transmissions occur at the same time. One synapse continues the impulse along a sensory neuron to the brain; the other immediately relays the impulse to an interneuron, which transmits it to a motor neuron.

The motor neuron delivers the impulse to a muscle or gland, producing an immediate response.

Cerebral cortex

Reflex arc
Interneuron
Dorsal root ganglion

Sensation
Sensory neuron

Reaction
Motor neuron

Incredibly Easy miniguide to physiology: Sound transmission

The illustration below details the transmission of sound through the structures of the middle and inner ear.

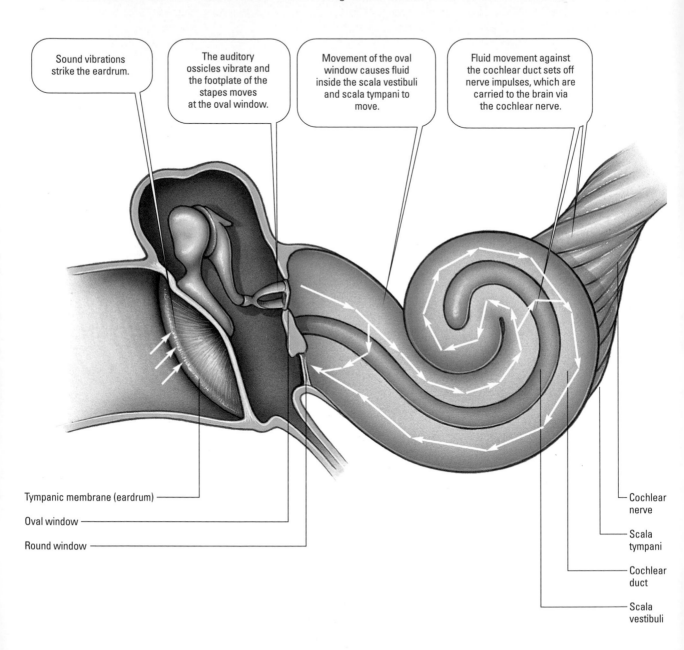

Sound vibrations strike the eardrum.

The auditory ossicles vibrate and the footplate of the stapes moves at the oval window.

Movement of the oval window causes fluid inside the scala vestibuli and scala tympani to move.

Fluid movement against the cochlear duct sets off nerve impulses, which are carried to the brain via the cochlear nerve.

Tympanic membrane (eardrum)

Oval window

Round window

Cochlear nerve

Scala tympani

Cochlear duct

Scala vestibuli

Incredibly Easy miniguide to physiology: The cardiac cycle

The cardiac cycle is the period from the beginning of one heartbeat to the beginning of the next. During this cycle, electrical and mechanical events must occur in the proper sequence and to the proper degree to provide adequate blood flow to all body parts. The cycle has two phases — systole and diastole.

Systole

At the beginning of systole, the ventricles contract, increasing pressure and forcing the mitral and tricuspid valves to close. As the ventricles contract, ventricular pressure builds up until it exceeds the pressure in the pulmonary artery and aorta. Then the aortic and pulmonic valves open, and the ventricles eject blood into the aorta and pulmonary artery.

Diastole

After the ventricles empty, they relax and ventricular pressure falls below that in the pulmonary artery and the aorta. At the beginning of diastole, the aortic and pulmonic valves close to prevent backflow of blood. During diastole, the mitral and tricuspid valves open and blood starts to flow into the ventricles from the atria.

Incredibly Easy miniguide to physiology: Cardiac conduction

The conduction system of the heart, shown below, begins with the heart's pacemaker, the sinoatrial (SA) node. When an impulse leaves the SA node, it travels through the atria along Bachmann's bundle and the internodal pathways on its way to the atrioventricular (AV) node and the ventricles. After the impulse passes through the AV node, it travels to the ventricles, first down the bundle of His, then along the bundle branches and, finally, down the Purkinje fibers.

Bachmann's bundle

SA node

Internodal tract
  Posterior (Thorel's)
  Middle (Wenckebach's)
  Anterior

AV node

Bundle of His

Right bundle branch

Left bundle branch

Purkinje fibers

This intricate system of conduction helps me keep my beat.

Incredibly Easy miniguide to physiology: Gas exchange

When the lungs fill with air, oxygen diffuses from the alveoli into the blood and carbon dioxide diffuses in the opposite direction. Gas exchange depends on differences in the partial pressures of the gases.

During inspiration, the partial pressure of water vapor increases, while partial pressures of the other gases decline. Before inspired air enters the alveoli, it mixes with gas that wasn't exhaled during the previous expiration. Because this gas contains more carbon dioxide and less oxygen than the inspired air, partial pressures change again.

Gas that enters the alveoli undergoes further partial pressure changes but retains a high P_{O_2} and a low P_{CO_2}. This gas meets deoxygenated blood from the right ventricle, which has a low P_{O_2} and a high P_{CO_2}. The pressure differential causes oxygen to diffuse into blood and carbon dioxide to diffuse out, equalizing gas pressures on both sides of the membrane.

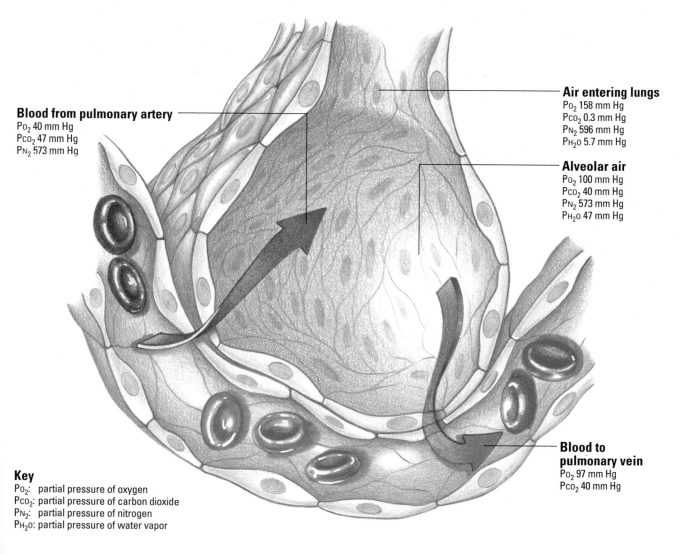

Air entering lungs
P_{O_2} 158 mm Hg
P_{CO_2} 0.3 mm Hg
P_{N_2} 596 mm Hg
P_{H_2O} 5.7 mm Hg

Alveolar air
P_{O_2} 100 mm Hg
P_{CO_2} 40 mm Hg
P_{N_2} 573 mm Hg
P_{H_2O} 47 mm Hg

Blood from pulmonary artery
P_{O_2} 40 mm Hg
P_{CO_2} 47 mm Hg
P_{N_2} 573 mm Hg

Blood to pulmonary vein
P_{O_2} 97 mm Hg
P_{CO_2} 40 mm Hg

Key
P_{O_2}: partial pressure of oxygen
P_{CO_2}: partial pressure of carbon dioxide
P_{N_2}: partial pressure of nitrogen
P_{H_2O}: partial pressure of water vapor

Incredibly Easy miniguide to physiology: Mechanics of ventilation

Breathing results from differences between atmospheric and intrapulmonary pressures, as described below.

 Before inspiration, intrapulmonary pressure equals atmospheric pressure (approximately 760 mm Hg). Intrapleural pressure is 756 mm Hg.

 During inspiration, the diaphragm and external intercostal muscles contract, enlarging the thorax vertically and horizontally. As the thorax expands, intrapleural pressure decreases and the lungs expand to fill the enlarging thoracic cavity.

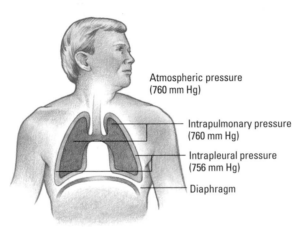

Atmospheric pressure
(760 mm Hg)

Intrapulmonary pressure
(760 mm Hg)

Intrapleural pressure
(756 mm Hg)

Diaphragm

Atmospheric pressure
(760 mm Hg)

Intrapulmonary pressure
(758 mm Hg)

Intrapleural pressure
(754 mm Hg)

 The intrapulmonary atmospheric pressure gradient pulls air into the lungs until the two pressures are equal.

 During normal expiration, the diaphragm slowly relaxes and the lungs and thorax passively return to resting size and position. During deep or forced expiration, contraction of internal intercostal and abdominal muscles reduces thoracic volume. Lung and thorax compression raises intrapulmonary pressure above atmospheric pressure.

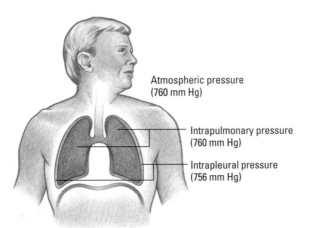

Atmospheric pressure
(760 mm Hg)

Intrapulmonary pressure
(760 mm Hg)

Intrapleural pressure
(756 mm Hg)

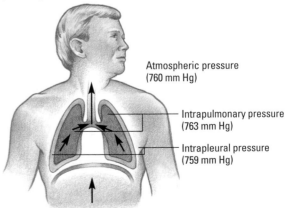

Atmospheric pressure
(760 mm Hg)

Intrapulmonary pressure
(763 mm Hg)

Intrapleural pressure
(759 mm Hg)

Incredibly Easy miniguide to physiology: Hormonal feedback mechanisms

Hypothalamic stimulation triggers a complex feedback mechanism that controls the blood levels of many hormones. First, the hypothalamus sends releasing and inhibiting factors or hormones to the anterior pituitary. In response, the anterior pituitary secretes tropic hormones, such as growth hormone (GH), prolactin (PRL), corticotropin, thyroid-stimulating hormone (TSH), follicle-stimulating hormone (FSH), and luteinizing hormone (LH). At the appropriate target gland, these hormones stimulate the target organ to release other hormones that regulate various body functions. When these hormones reach normal levels in body tissue, a feedback mechanism inhibits further hypothalamic and pituitary secretion.

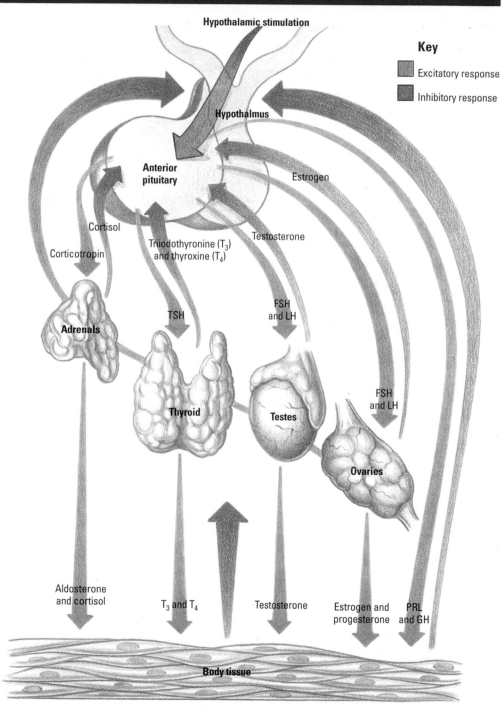

Key

Excitatory response

Inhibitory response

Hypothalamic stimulation

Hypothalmus

Anterior pituitary

Estrogen

Cortisol

Testosterone

Corticotropin

Triiodothyronine (T_3) and thyroxine (T_4)

TSH

FSH and LH

Adrenals

Thyroid

Testes

FSH and LH

Ovaries

Aldosterone and cortisol

T_3 and T_4

Testosterone

Estrogen and progesterone

PRL and GH

Body tissue

Incredibly Easy miniguide to physiology: Hormone storage and release

Endocrine cells manufacture and release their hormones in several ways, as described here.

Pancreas

Many endocrine cells possess receptors on their membranes that respond to stimuli:
- Neuron stimulation of pancreatic beta cells (shown at right) causes production of the hormone precursor preproinsulin.
- Preproinsulin is converted to proinsulin in beadlike ribosomes located on the endoplasmic reticulum.
- Proinsulin is transferred to the Golgi complex, which collects it into secretory granules and converts it to insulin.
- Secretory granules fuse with the plasma membrane and disperse insulin into the bloodstream.
- Hormonal release by membrane fusion is called *exocytosis*.

Nucleus
Neural synapse
Preproinsulin
Granular endoplasmic reticulum
Ribosome
Proinsulin

Insulin
Capillary lumen
Secretory granules (containing insulin)
Mitochondrion
Golgi complex
Plasma membrane

Thyroid

Thyroid cells store a hormone precursor, colloidal iodinated thyroglobulin, which contains iodine and thyroglobulin. When stimulated by thyroid-stimulating hormone (TSH), a follicular cell (shown at right) takes up some stored thyroglobulin by *endocytosis*—the reverse of exocytosis.

The cell membrane extends fingerlike projections into the colloid, and then pulls portions of it back into the cell. Lysosomes fuse with the colloid, which is then degraded into triiodothyronine (T_3) and thyroxine (T_4). These thyroid hormones are released into the circulation and lymphatic system by exocytosis.

Colloidal iodinated thyroglobulin
Iodine
Thyroglobulin secretion
Lysosome
Blood vessel lumen
T_3 and T_4
TSH
Amino acids
Iodide
T_3 and T_4
Lymph vessel lumen

Incredibly Easy miniguide to physiology: Hormone storage and release

Hypothalamus and pituitary

Anterior and posterior pituitary secretions are controlled by signals from the hypothalamus:

• As shown on the left side of the illustration at right, the hypothalamic neuron produces antidiuretic hormone (ADH), which travels down the axon and is stored in secretory granules in nerve endings in the posterior pituitary for later release.

• As shown on the right side of the illustration at right, the hypothalamus stimulates the anterior pituitary's production of its many hormones. A hypothalamic neuron manufactures inhibitory and stimulatory hormones and secretes them into a capillary of the portal system. The hormones travel down the pituitary stalk to the anterior pituitary. There, they cause inhibition or release of many pituitary hormones, including corticotropin, TSH, growth hormone, follicle-stimulating hormone, luteinizing hormone, and prolactin.

Different types of hormones are controlled by different endocrine cells. For example, pituitary secretions are controlled by the hypothalamus.

Incredibly Easy miniguide to physiology: Membrane transport mechanisms

Substances move across a cell membrane either by passive or active transport mechanisms. They can enter or leave a cell by passing through the cell membrane or by moving through pores in the protein molecules embedded in the membrane.

Passive transport
No energy is required for passive transport. It occurs through two mechanisms: diffusion and osmosis.

Diffusion
In diffusion, substances move from an area of higher concentration to an area of lower concentration. Movement continues until distribution is uniform.

Osmosis
In osmosis, water molecules move from an area of higher concentration to one of lower concentration.

Diffusion

Cell membrane

Substance

Osmosis

Cell membrane

Water

No energy is required for passive transport. And it's a good thing because I have my hands full already!

Incredibly Easy miniguide to physiology: Membrane transport mechanisms

Active transport

Active transport moves molecules and ions against a concentration gradient from an area of lower concentration to one of higher concentration. This movement requires energy, usually in the form of adenosine triphosphate (ATP). The sodium-potassium pump and pinocytosis are examples of active transport mechanisms.

Sodium-potassium pump

The sodium-potassium pump moves sodium from inside the cell to outside, where the sodium concentration is greater; potassium moves from outside the cell to inside, where the potassium concentration is greater.

Pinocytosis

In pinocytosis, tiny vacuoles take droplets of fluid containing dissolved substances into the cell. The engulfed fluid is used in the cell.

Sodium-potassium pump

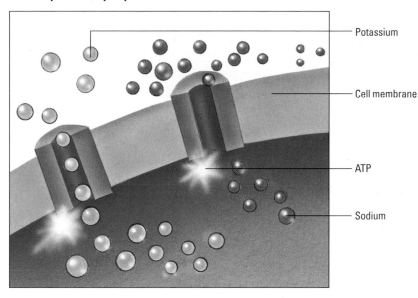

- Potassium
- Cell membrane
- ATP
- Sodium

Pinocytosis

- Cell membrane
- Fluid with dissolved substances
- Vacuole

Energy is needed for active transport.

Incredibly Easy miniguide: Renin-angiotensin-aldosterone system

The renin-angiotensin-aldosterone system regulates the body's sodium and water levels and blood pressure. Juxtaglomerular cells (1) near the glomeruli in each kidney secrete the enzyme renin into the blood.

Renin circulates throughout the body and converts angiotensinogen, made in the liver (2), into angiotensin I. In the lungs (3), angiotensin I is converted by hydrolysis to angiotensin II. Angiotensin II acts on the adrenal cortex (4) to stimulate production of the hormone aldosterone. Aldosterone acts on the juxtaglomerular cells to increase sodium and water retention and to stimulate or depress further renin secretion, completing the feedback system that automatically readjusts homeostasis.

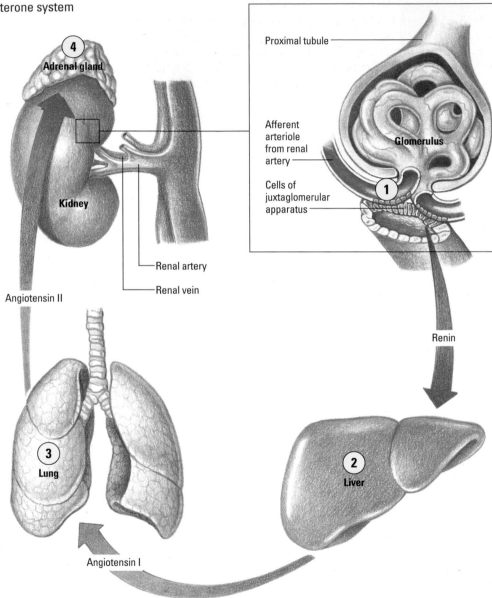

Proximal tubule

Glomerulus

Afferent arteriole from renal artery

Cells of juxtaglomerular apparatus

1

4
Adrenal gland

Kidney

Renal artery

Renal vein

Angiotensin II

Renin

3
Lung

2
Liver

Angiotensin I

Incredibly Easy miniguide to physiology: The menstrual cycle

The hypothalamus, ovaries, and pituitary gland secrete hormones that effect the buildup and shedding of the endometrium during the menstrual cycle. The menstrual cycle normally occurs over 28 days, although it may range from 22 to 34 days. The cycle is regulated by fluctuating hormone levels that, in turn, are regulated by negative and positive feedback mechanisms involving the hypothalamus, pituitary glands, and ovaries.

The hormonal changes of the menstrual cycle trigger a series of changes in the uterine endometrium as follows:
• menstrual (preovulatory) phase—endometrium exfoliates and sheds
• proliferative (follicular) phase and ovulation—endometrium proliferates
• luteal (secretory) phase—endometrium becomes thick and secretory to prepare for the implantation of a fertilized ovum
• premenstrual phase—in absence of fertilization, estrogen and progesterone levels drop and the endometrium sheds.

These illustrations show the relationship between ovarian changes and uterine changes during the menstrual cycle.

Ovary

Primary oocyte | Developing follicles | Mature graafian follicle | Antrum filled with liquor folliculi | Expulsion of the secondary oocyte | Corpus luteum of menstruation

Uterus

Ovulation

Endometrium

Stratum functionale

Stratum basale

Myometrium

Uterine gland

Venous lacunae

Endometrial vein

Spiral artery
Basal artery

Arcuate artery

Day 0   4   14   26   28

Menstrual phase | **Proliferative phase** | **Secretory phase** | **Premenstrual phase**

Incredibly Easy miniguide to physiology: Fertilization and implantation

During monthly ovulation, an ovum is released from the ovary into the fallopian tube, where it travels toward the uterus. If present, sperm from the male move through the fallopian tube, where they meet the ovum.

If a sperm penetrates the ovum, fertilization occurs and the ovum is called a *zygote.* The zygote continues to travel toward the uterus, dividing many times until it becomes a blastocyst. When the blastocyst reaches the uterus, it implants in the uterine wall and continues to develop over the next nine months.

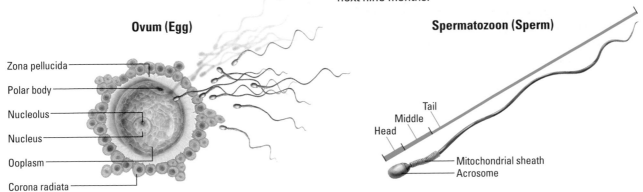

Ovum (Egg)

Zona pellucida
Polar body
Nucleolus
Nucleus
Ooplasm
Corona radiata

Spermatozoon (Sperm)

Tail
Middle
Head
Mitochondrial sheath
Acrosome

Fertilization and implantation

Early cell division of zygote

Two-cell stage
Four-cell stage
Eight-cell stage
Morula
Implanted blastocyst
Fertilization
Ovum
Corpus luteum
Ovarian ligament
Fallopian tube
Infundibulum
Fimbria
Ovary
Vesicular appendix
Uterus
Mucus plug
Cervix
Vagina

Incredibly easy miniguide to physiology: Inflammatory response

The inflammatory response helps the body return to homeostasis after a wound occurs. Its primary function is to bring phagocytic cells (neutrophils and monocytes) to the inflamed area to destroy bacteria and rid the tissue spaces of dead and dying cells so that tissue repair can begin.

Inflammation produces four cardinal signs: redness, swelling, heat, and pain. The first three signs result from local vasodilation, fluid leakage into the extravascular space, and blockage of lymphatic drainage. The fourth results from tissue space distention caused by swelling and pressure and from chemical irritation of nociceptors (pain receptors).

Epidermis

Dermis

Blood vessel

(1) Splinter punctures epidermis

(2) Bacteria introduced

(3) Bacteria implanted in tissue

(4) Injured cells release histamine and kinins, causing capillary dilation

(5) Dilated capillaries make skin hot and red; escaping fluid from blood vessels causes swelling; edema, kinins, and other substances produce pain; phagocytes migrate through vessel walls toward bacteria

(6) Neutrophils and monocytes destroy bacteria by phagocytosis

Incredibly Easy miniguide: Immune response to bacterial invasion

Invasion of a foreign substance can trigger two types of immune responses — antibody-mediated (humoral) and cell-mediated immunity:

• In *humoral* immunity, antigens stimulate B cells to differentiate into plasma cells and produce circulating antibodies that disable bacteria and viruses before they can enter host cells.

• In *cell-mediated* immunity, T cells move directly to attack invaders. Three T-cell subgroups trigger the response to infection. Helper T cells spur B cells to manufacture antibodies. Effector T cells kill antigens and produce lymphokines (proteins that induce inflammatory response and mediate the delayed hypersensitivity reaction). Suppressor T cells regulate T and B types of immune response.

In cell-mediated immunity, I'm on guard, ready to attack invaders.

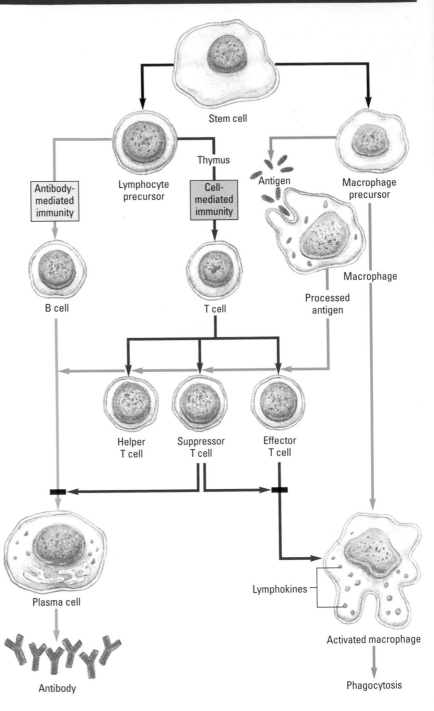

Stem cell

Lymphocyte precursor

Thymus

Antibody-mediated immunity

Cell-mediated immunity

Antigen

Macrophage precursor

B cell

T cell

Macrophage

Processed antigen

Helper T cell

Suppressor T cell

Effector T cell

Plasma cell

Lymphokines

Antibody

Activated macrophage

Phagocytosis

Now I get it!

How aldosterone works

Here's how aldosterone acts to regulate fluid volume.

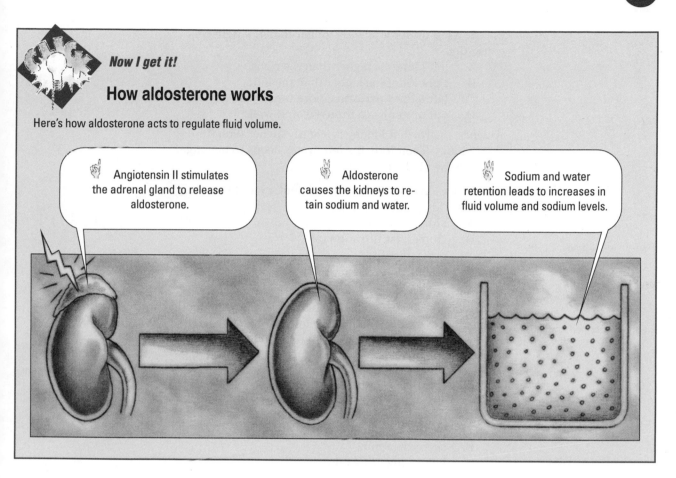

Angiotensin II stimulates the adrenal gland to release aldosterone.

Aldosterone causes the kidneys to retain sodium and water.

Sodium and water retention leads to increases in fluid volume and sodium levels.

Quick quiz

1. In a normal adult, bladder capacity ranges from:
   A. 50 to 100 ml.
   B. 200 to 300 ml.
   C. 500 to 600 ml.
   D. 700 to 900 ml.

Answer: C. In a normal adult, bladder capacity ranges from 500 to 600 ml.

2. The left ureter is slightly longer than the right because the:

    A.   left kidney is higher than the right.
    B.   right kidney is higher than the left.
    C.   left kidney performs more functions.
    D.   left ureter has a three-layered wall.

Answer: A. The left kidney is slightly higher than the right kidney. Therefore, the left ureter needs to be longer to reach the bladder.

3. Urination results from an involuntary and voluntary process. This process is called the:

    A.   kidney process.
    B.   glomerular filtration rate.
    C.   prostate reflex.
    D.   micturition reflex.

Answer: D. The micturition reflex is the signal system that occurs when urine fills the bladder. Parasympathetic nerve fibers in the bladder wall cause the bladder to contract and the internal sphincter to relax, which is followed by a voluntary relaxation of the external sphincter.

4. A person on a new health regimen has begun to drink at least 8 oz (236 ml) of water six to eight times per day. The kidneys react to this change by:

    A.   producing aldosterone.
    B.   secreting renin.
    C.   increasing urine output.
    D.   secreting erythropoietin.

Answer: C. Urine output typically varies with fluid intake and climate. After ingestion of a large volume of fluid, urine output increases as the body rapidly excretes excess water.

Scoring

☆☆☆ If you answered all four questions correctly, congratulations! You've got the kidneys (and ureters, bladder, and urethra) down cold.

☆☆ If you answered three questions correctly, not bad! You're learning to navigate the urinary system.

☆ If you answered fewer than three questions correctly, be of good cheer. There's still ample time for you to become an expert on anatomy and physiology!

15

Fluids, electrolytes, acids, and bases

Just the facts

In this chapter, you'll learn:

♦ the way in which fluids are distributed throughout the body

♦ the kidneys' role in electrolyte balance

♦ the body's way of compensating for acid-base imbalances

♦ major acid-base imbalances.

Fluid balance

The health and *homeostasis* (equilibrium of the various body functions) of the human body depend on *fluid*, *electrolyte*, and *acid-base balance*. Factors that disrupt this balance, such as surgery, illness, and injury, can lead to potentially fatal changes in metabolic activity. (See *How the body gains and loses fluids*, page 250.)

Fluids, electrolytes, acids, and bases — it's a balancing act to keep the body functioning correctly.

Body shop

How the body gains and loses fluids

Each day, the body takes in fluid from the GI tract (in foods, liquids, and water of oxidation) and loses fluids through the skin, lungs, intestines (stool), and urinary tract (urine). This illustration shows the primary sites involved in fluid gains and losses as well as the amount of normal daily fluid intake and output.

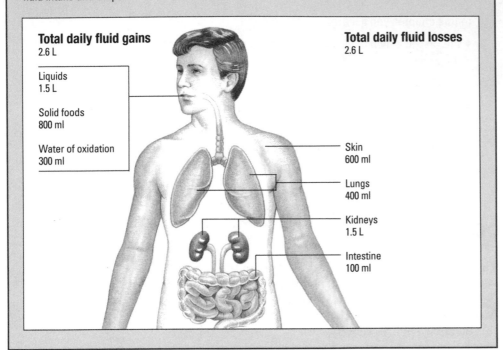

Total daily fluid gains
2.6 L

Liquids
1.5 L

Solid foods
800 ml

Water of oxidation
300 ml

Total daily fluid losses
2.6 L

Skin
600 ml

Lungs
400 ml

Kidneys
1.5 L

Intestine
100 ml

The four fluids

Body fluid is made up of water containing *solutes*, or dissolved substances, that are necessary for physiologic functioning. Solutes include electrolytes, glucose, amino acids, and other nutrients. There are four types of body fluids:

• *Intracellular fluid (ICF)* is found within the individual cells of the body.

• *Intravascular fluid (IVF)* is found within the plasma and the lymphatic system.

• *Interstitial fluid (ISF)* is found in the loose tissue around cells.

Water weight

Water in the body exists in two major compartments that are separated by capillary walls and cell membranes. About two-thirds of the body's water is found within cells as intracellular fluid (ICF); the other third remains outside cells as extracellular fluid (ECF).

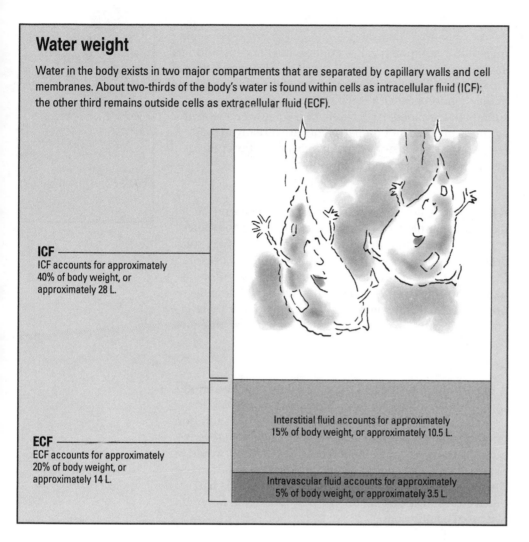

ICF
ICF accounts for approximately 40% of body weight, or approximately 28 L.

ECF
ECF accounts for approximately 20% of body weight, or approximately 14 L.

Interstitial fluid accounts for approximately 15% of body weight, or approximately 10.5 L.

Intravascular fluid accounts for approximately 5% of body weight, or approximately 3.5 L.

• *Extracellular fluid (ECF),* found in the spaces between cells, includes IVF and ISF.

Playing the percentages

ICF and ECF comprise about 40% and 20%, respectively, of an adult's total body weight. (See *Water weight.*)

Fluid forms and movement

Fluids in the body generally aren't found in pure forms. They're most commonly found in three different types of solutions: isotonic, hypotonic, and hypertonic.

No shifting needed

An isotonic solution has the same solute concentration as another solution. For example, normal saline solution is considered isotonic because the concentration of sodium in the solution is nearly equal to the concentration of sodium in the blood. As a result, two equally concentrated fluids in adjacent compartments are already in balance so the fluid inside each compartment stays put; no imbalance means no net fluid shift.

Memory jogger

To help remember which fluid belongs to which compartment, keep in mind that *inter* means *between* (as in "interval") and *intra* means *within* or *inside* (as in "intravenous").

Go low for hypo...

A hypotonic solution has a lower solute concentration than another solution. For instance, when one solution contains less sodium than another solution, the first solution is hypotonic compared with the second. As a result, fluid from the first solution — the hypotonic solution — would shift into the second solution until the two solutions had equal concentrations. (Remember, the body constantly strives to maintain a state of balance, or equilibrium.)

...and high for hyper

A hypertonic solution has a higher solute concentration than another solution. For instance, when one solution contains a large amount of sodium and a second solution contains hardly any, the first solution is hypertonic compared with the second solution. As a result, fluid would be drawn from the second solution into the first solution — the hypertonic solution — until the two solutions had equal concentrations. Again, the body strives to maintain a state of equilibrium.

Fluid movement within the cells

Just as the heart beats constantly, fluids and solutes move constantly within the body. That movement allows the body to maintain *homeostasis*, the constant state of balance the body seeks.

Solutes within the various compartments of the body (intracellular, interstitial, and intravascular) move through the membranes that separate those compartments. The membranes are semipermeable, meaning that they allow some solutes to pass through but not others. Solutes move through membranes at the cellular level by diffusion (movement of particles from an area of high concentration to an area of lower concentration), active transport, or osmosis.

Upstream...

In *active transport*, solutes move from an area of lower concentration to an area of higher concentration. Think of active transport as swimming upstream. When a fish swims upstream, it has to expend energy.

...and against the current

The energy required for a solute to move against a concentration gradient comes from a substance called *adenosine triphosphate (ATP)*. Stored in all cells, ATP supplies energy for solute movement in and out of cells.

Some solutes, such as sodium and potassium, use ATP to move in and out of cells in a form of active transport called the *sodium-potassium pump*. Other solutes that require active transport to cross cell membranes include calcium ions, hydrogen ions, amino acids, and certain sugars.

Just passing through

Osmosis refers to the passive movement of fluid across a membrane from an area of lower solute concentration and comparatively more fluid into an area of higher solute concentration and comparatively less fluid. Osmosis stops when enough fluid has moved through the membrane to equalize the solute concentration on both sides of the membrane.

In with the good

Water normally enters the body from the GI tract. Each day, the body obtains about 1.6 qt (1.5 L) of water from consumed liquids and approximately 26.6 oz (800 ml) more from solid foods, which may consist of up to 97% water. Oxidation of food in the body yields carbon dioxide (CO_2) and about 10 oz (300 ml) of water (water of oxidation).

Out with the bad

Water leaves the body through the skin (in perspiration), lungs (in expired air), GI tract (in stool), and urinary tract (in urine).

The major pipeline

The main route of water loss is urine excretion, which typically varies from 1 to 2.6 L daily. Water losses through the skin (600 ml) and lungs (400 ml) amount to 1 L daily but may increase markedly with strenuous exertion, which predisposes a person to dehydration.

Don't interrupt

In a healthy body, fluid gains match fluid losses to maintain proper physiologic functioning. However, interruption or dysfunction of one or both of the mechanisms that regulate fluid balance — thirst and the *countercurrent mechanism* — can lead to a fluid imbalance.

I'm parched!

Thirst — the conscious desire for water — is the primary regulator of fluid intake. When the body becomes dehydrated, ECF volume is reduced, causing an increase in sodium concentration and osmolarity.

When the sodium concentration reaches about 2 mEq/L above normal, neurons of the thirst center in the hypothalamus are stimulated. The brain then directs motor neurons to satisfy thirst, causing the person to drink enough fluid to restore ECF to normal.

What comes in must go out

Through the countercurrent mechanism, the kidneys regulate fluid output by modifying urine concentration — that is, by excreting urine of greater or lesser concentration, depending on fluid balance.

Electrolyte balance

Electrolytes are substances that *dissociate* (break up) into electrically charged particles, called *ions*, when dissolved in water. Adequate amounts of each major electrolyte and a proper balance among the electrolytes are required to maintain normal physiologic functioning.

All charged up

Ions may be positively charged (called *cations*) or negatively charged (called *anions*). Major cations include sodium, potassium, calcium, and magnesium. Major anions include chloride, bicarbonate (HCO_3^-), and phosphate.

Normally, the electrical charges of cations balance the electrical charges of anions, keeping body fluids electrically neutral. Blood plasma contains slightly more electrolytes than does ISF.

Shh! We're concentrating

Because ions are present in such low concentrations in body fluids, they're usually expressed in milliequivalents per liter (mEq/L). ICF and ECF cells are permeable to different substances; therefore, these compartments normally have different electrolyte compositions. (See *Electrolyte composition in ICF and ECF.*)

A delicate balance

Electrolytes profoundly affect the body's water distribution, osmolarity, and acid-base balance. Numerous mechanisms within the body help maintain electrolyte balance. Dysfunction or interruption of any of these mechanisms can produce an electrolyte imbalance.

Electrolyte composition in ICF and ECF

This chart shows the electrolyte compositions of intracellular fluid (ICF) and extracellular fluid (ECF).

Electrolyte	ICF	ECF
Sodium	10 mEq/L	136 to 146 mEq/L
Potassium	140 mEq/L	3.6 to 5 mEq/L
Calcium	10 mEq/L	4.5 to 5.8 mEq/L
Magnesium	40 mEq/L	1.6 to 2.2 mEq/L
Chloride	4 mEq/L	96 to 106 mEq/L
Bicarbonate	10 mEq/L	24 to 28 mEq/L
Phosphate	100 mEq/L	1 to 1.5 mEq/L

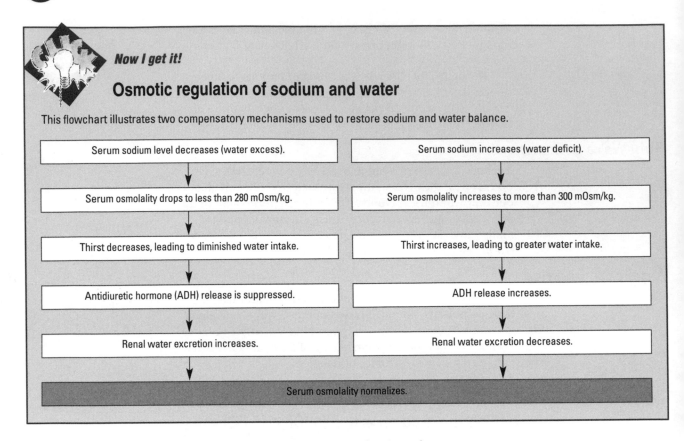

Now I get it!

Osmotic regulation of sodium and water

This flowchart illustrates two compensatory mechanisms used to restore sodium and water balance.

Serum sodium level decreases (water excess).	Serum sodium increases (water deficit).
↓	↓
Serum osmolality drops to less than 280 mOsm/kg.	Serum osmolality increases to more than 300 mOsm/kg.
↓	↓
Thirst decreases, leading to diminished water intake.	Thirst increases, leading to greater water intake.
↓	↓
Antidiuretic hormone (ADH) release is suppressed.	ADH release increases.
↓	↓
Renal water excretion increases.	Renal water excretion decreases.

Serum osmolality normalizes.

Here are the regulatory mechanisms for common electrolytes:

• The kidneys and a hormone called *aldosterone* are the chief sodium regulators. The small intestine absorbs sodium readily from food, and the skin and kidneys excrete sodium. (See *Osmotic regulation of sodium and water.*)

• The kidneys also regulate potassium through aldosterone action. Most potassium is absorbed from food in the GI tract; normally, the amount excreted in urine equals dietary potassium intake.

• Calcium in the blood is typically in equilibrium with calcium salts in bone. Parathyroid hormone (PTH) is the main regulator of calcium, controlling both calcium uptake from the GI tract and calcium excretion by the kidneys.

• Magnesium is governed by aldosterone, which controls renal magnesium reabsorption. Absorbed from the GI tract, magnesium is excreted in urine, breast milk, and saliva.

• The kidneys also regulate chloride. Chloride ions move in conjunction with sodium ions.
• The kidneys regulate HCO_3^-, excreting, absorbing, or forming it. HCO_3^-, in turn, plays a vital part in acid-base balance.
• The kidneys regulate phosphate. Absorbed from food, phosphate is incorporated with calcium in bone. PTH governs calcium and phosphate levels.

I'm an electrolyte superstar — helping to regulate potassium, chloride, bicarbonate, and phosphate.

Acid-base balance

Physiologic survival requires *acid-base balance*, a stable concentration of hydrogen ions in body fluids.

An acid remark

An *acid* is a substance that yields hydrogen ions when *dissociated* (changed from a complex to a simpler compound) in solution. A strong acid dissociates almost completely, releasing a large number of hydrogen ions.

A base reply

A *base* dissociates in water, releasing ions that can combine with hydrogen ions. Like a strong acid, a strong base dissociates almost completely, releasing many ions.

The hydrogen ion concentration of a fluid determines whether it's *acidic* or *basic* (alkaline). A *neutral* solution, such as pure water, dissociates only slightly. (See *Understanding pH*, page 258.)

Keep those ions coming

The body produces acids, thus yielding hydrogen ions, through the following mechanisms:
• Protein catabolism yields nonvolatile acids, such as sulfuric, phosphoric, and uric acids.
• Fat oxidation produces acid ketone bodies.
• Anaerobic glucose catabolism produces lactic acid.
• Intracellular metabolism yields CO_2 as a by-product; CO_2 dissolves in body fluids to form carbonic acid (H_2CO_3).

Will a fluid be acidic or basic? Only the hydrogen ion concentration knows for sure.

Balancing buffers

Normally, even with the production of these acids, the body's pH control mechanism is so effective that blood pH stays within a narrow

Now I get it!

Understanding pH

Hydrogen (H) ion concentration is commonly expressed as pH, which indicates the degree of acidity or alkalinity of a solution:
• A pH of 7 indicates neutrality or equal amounts of H and hydroxyl (OH^-) ions.
• An acidic solution contains more H ions than OH^- ions; its pH is less than 7.
• An alkaline solution contains fewer H ions than OH^- ions; its pH exceeds 7.
    Overall, as H ion concentration increases, pH goes down.

1 means 10
Because pH is an exponential expression, a change of one pH unit reflects a 10-fold difference in actual H ion concentration. For instance, a solution with a pH of 7 has 10 times more H ions than a solution with a pH of 8.

range: 7.35 to 7.45. This acid-base balance is maintained by buffer systems and the lungs and kidneys, which neutralize and eliminate acids as rapidly as they're formed.

Dysfunction or interruption of a buffer system or other governing mechanism can cause an acid-base imbalance. (See *Understanding respiratory and metabolic alkalosis and acidosis.*)

Buffer systems

Buffer systems reduce the effect of an abrupt change in hydrogen ion concentration by converting a strong acid or base (which normally would dissociate completely) into a weak acid or base (which releases fewer hydrogen ions).

Buffer systems that help maintain acid-base balance include:
• sodium bicarbonate–carbonic acid
• phosphate
• protein.

(Text continues on page 263.)

Now I get it!

Understanding respiratory and metabolic alkalosis and acidosis

What happens in respiratory alkalosis

Step 1

When pulmonary ventilation increases above the amount needed to maintain normal carbon dioxide (CO_2) levels, excessive amounts of CO_2 are exhaled. This causes hypocapnia (a fall in partial pressure of arterial carbon dioxide [$Paco_2$]), which leads to a reduction in carbonic acid (H_2CO_3) production, a loss of hydrogen (H) ions and bicarbonate (HCO_3^-) ions, and a subsequent rise in pH. Look for a pH level above 7.45, a $Paco_2$ level below 35 mm Hg, and an HCO_3^- level below 22 mEq/L (as shown at right).

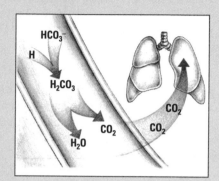

Step 2

In defense against the rising pH, H ions are pulled out of the cells and into the blood in exchange for potassium (K) ions. The H ions entering the blood combine with HCO_3^- ions to form H_2CO_3, which lowers the pH. Look for a further decrease in HCO_3^- levels, a fall in pH, and a fall in serum K levels (hypokalemia).

Step 3

Hypocapnia stimulates the carotid and aortic bodies and the medulla, which causes an increase in heart rate without an increase in blood pressure (as shown at right). Look for angina, electrocardiogram changes, restlessness, and anxiety.

Step 4

Simultaneously, hypocapnia produces cerebral vasoconstriction, which prompts a reduction in cerebral blood flow. Hypocapnia also overexcites the medulla, pons, and other parts of the autonomic nervous system. Look for increasing anxiety, diaphoresis, dyspnea, alternating periods of apnea and hyperventilation, dizziness, and tingling in the fingers or toes.

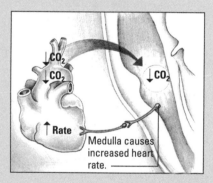

Step 5

When hypocapnia lasts more than 6 hours, the kidneys increase secretion of HCO_3^- and reduce excretion of H (as shown at right). Periods of apnea may result if the pH remains high and the $Paco_2$ remains low. Look for slowing of the respiratory rate, hypoventilation, and Cheyne-Stokes respirations.

Step 6

Continued low $Paco_2$ increases cerebral and peripheral hypoxia from vasoconstriction. Severe alkalosis inhibits calcium (Ca) ionization which, in turn, causes increased nerve excitability and muscle contractions. Eventually, the alkalosis overwhelms the central nervous system (CNS) and the heart. Look for decreasing level of consciousness (LOC), hyperreflexia, carpopedal spasm, tetany, arrhythmias, seizures, and coma.

(continued)

Understanding respiratory and metabolic alkalosis and acidosis (continued)

What happens in respiratory acidosis

Step 1

When pulmonary ventilation decreases, retained CO_2 combines with water (H_2O) to form H_2CO_3 in larger-than-normal amounts. The H_2CO_3 dissociates to release free H and HCO_3^- ions. The excessive H_2CO_3 causes a drop in pH. Look for a $Paco_2$ level above 45 mm Hg and a pH level below 7.35.

Step 2

As the pH level falls, 2,3-diphosphoglycerate (2,3-DPG) increases in the red blood cells and causes a change in hemoglobin (Hb) that makes the Hb release oxygen (O_2). The altered Hb, now strongly alkaline, picks up H ions and CO_2, thus eliminating some of the free H ions and excess CO_2 (as shown at right). Look for decreased arterial oxygen saturation.

Step 3

Whenever $Paco_2$ increases, CO_2 builds up in all tissues and fluids, including cerebrospinal fluid and the respiratory center in the medulla. The CO_2 reacts with H_2O to form H_2CO_3, which then breaks into free H and HCO_3^- ions. The increased amount of CO_2 and free H ions stimulate the respiratory center to increase the respiratory rate. An increased respiratory rate expels more CO_2 and helps to reduce the CO_2 level in the blood and other tissues. Look for rapid, shallow respirations and a decreasing $Paco_2$.

Step 4

Eventually, CO_2 and H ions cause cerebral blood vessels to dilate, which increases blood flow to the brain. That increased flow can cause cerebral edema and depress CNS activity. Look for headache, confusion, lethargy, nausea, or vomiting. As respiratory mechanisms fail, the increasing $Paco_2$ stimulates the kidneys to retain HCO_3^- and sodium (Na) ions and to excrete H ions, some of which are excreted in the form of ammonium (NH_4). The additional HCO_3^- and Na combine to form extra sodium bicarbonate ($NaHCO_3^-$), which is then able to buffer more free H ions (as shown at right). Look for increased acid content in the urine, increasing serum pH and HCO_3^- levels, and shallow, depressed respirations.

Step 5

As the concentration of H ions overwhelms the body's compensatory mechanisms, the H ions move into the cells and K ions move out. A concurrent lack of O_2 causes an increase in the anaerobic production of lactic acid, which further skews the acid-base balance and critically depresses neurologic and cardiac functions. Look for hyperkalemia, arrhythmias, increased $Paco_2$, decreased partial pressure of arterial oxygen, decreased pH, and decreased LOC.

Understanding respiratory and metabolic alkalosis and acidosis *(continued)*

What happens in metabolic alkalosis

Step 1

As HCO_3^- ions start to accumulate in the body, chemical buffers (in extracellular fluid [ECF] and cells) bind with the ions. No signs are detectable at this stage.

Step 2

Excess HCO_3^- ions that don't bind with chemical buffers elevate serum pH levels, which, in turn, depress chemoreceptors in the medulla. Depression of those chemoreceptors causes a decrease in respiratory rate, which increases the $Paco_2$. The additional CO_2 combines with H_2O to form H_2CO_3 (as shown at right). Note: Lowered O_2 levels limit respiratory compensation. Look for a serum pH level above 7.45, an HCO_3^- level above 26 mEq/L, a rising $Paco_2$, and slow, shallow respirations.

Step 3

When the HCO_3^- level exceeds 28 mEq/L, the renal glomeruli can no longer reabsorb excess HCO_3^-. That excess HCO_3^- is excreted in the urine; H ions are retained. Look for alkaline urine and pH and HCO_3^- levels that slowly return to normal.

Step 4

To maintain electrochemical balance, the kidneys excrete excess Na ions, H_2O, and HCO_3^- (as shown at right). Look for polyuria initially, and then signs of hypovolemia, including thirst and dry mucous membranes.

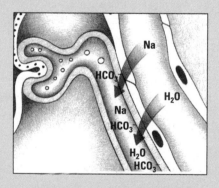

Step 5

Lowered H ion levels in the ECF cause the ions to diffuse out of the cells. To maintain the balance of charge across the cell membrane, extracellular K ions move into the cells. Look for signs of hypokalemia: anorexia, muscle weakness, loss of reflexes, and others.

Step 6

As H ion levels decline, Ca ionization decreases. That decrease in ionization makes nerve cells more permeable to Na ions. Na ions moving into nerve cells stimulate neural impulses and produce overexcitability of the peripheral nervous system and CNS. Look for tetany, belligerence, irritability, disorientation, and seizures.

> Metabolic alkalosis ultimately progresses to tetany, belligerence, irritability, disorientation, and seizures.

(continued)

Understanding respiratory and metabolic alkalosis and acidosis *(continued)*

What happens in metabolic acidosis

Step 1
As H ions start to accumulate in the body, chemical buffers (plasma HCO_3^- and proteins) in the cells and ECF bind with them (as shown at right). No signs are detectable at this stage.

Chemical buffer

Step 2
Excess H ions (which can't bind with the buffers) decrease the pH and stimulate chemoreceptors in the medulla to increase the respiratory rate. The increased respiratory rate lowers the $Paco_2$, which allows more H ions to bind with HCO_3^- ions. Respiratory compensation occurs within minutes, but isn't sufficient to correct the imbalance (see middle illustration). Look for a pH level below 7.35, an HCO_3^- level below 22 mEq/L, a decreasing $Paco_2$ level, and rapid, deeper respirations.

Step 3
Healthy kidneys try to compensate for the acidosis by secreting excess H ions into the renal tubules. Those ions are buffered by phosphate or ammonia and then are excreted into the urine in the form of a weak acid. Look for acidic urine.

Step 4
Each time an H ion is secreted into the renal tubules, an Na ion and an HCO_3^- ion are absorbed from the tubules and returned to the blood. Look for pH and HCO_3^- levels that slowly return to normal.

Step 5
Excess H ions in the ECF diffuse into cells. To maintain the balance of the charge across the membrane, the cells release K ions into the blood (as shown at right). Look for signs of hyperkalemia, including colic and diarrhea, weakness or flaccid paralysis, tingling and numbness in the extremities, bradycardia, a tall T wave, a prolonged PR interval, and a wide QRS complex.

Step 6
Excess H ions alter the normal balance of K, Na, and Ca ions, leading to reduced excitability of nerve cells. Look for signs and symptoms of progressive CNS depression, including lethargy, dull headache, confusion, stupor, and coma.

One from the kidneys, one from the lungs

The *sodium bicarbonate–carbonic acid* buffer system is the major buffer in ECF. Sodium bicarbonate ($NaHCO_3^-$) concentration is regulated by the kidneys, and H_2CO_3 concentration is regulated by the lungs. Both components of this buffer are replenished continually. As a result of the buffering action, the strong base (sodium hydroxide [NaOH]) is replaced by $NaHCO_3^-$ and water (H_2O). NaOH dissociates almost completely and releases large amounts of hydroxyl (OH^-). If a strong acid is added, the opposite occurs.

> We team up to keep blood pH normal — between 7.35 and 7.45.

Finesse with phosphate

A *phosphate* buffer system works by regulating the pH of fluids as they pass through the kidneys. It's also important in ECF. Its acidic component is *sodium dihydrogen phosphate* (NaH_2PO_4); its alkaline component is *sodium monohydrogen phosphate* (Na_2HPO_4).

Absorbing ions

Protein buffers can exist in the form of acids or alkaline salts. In the *protein* buffer system, intracellular proteins absorb hydrogen (H^+) ions generated by the body's metabolic processes and may release excess H^+ as needed.

Lungs

The protein buffer system changes the pH of the blood in 3 minutes or less by changing the breathing rate. A decreased respiratory rate decreases the exchange and release of CO_2, there is less H^+, and the pH rises. Present in all acids, H ions are protons that can be added to or removed from a solution to change the pH.

Respiration plays a crucial role in controlling pH. The lungs excrete CO_2 and regulate the H_2CO_3 content of the blood. H_2CO_3 is derived from the CO_2 and H_2O that are released as by-products of cellular metabolic activity.

Stick to the formula

CO_2 is soluble in blood plasma. Some of the dissolved gas reacts with H_2O to form H_2CO_3, a weak acid that partially breaks apart to form H and HCO_3^- ions. These three substances are in equilibrium, as reflected in the following formula:

$$CO_2 + H_2O \leftrightarrow H_2CO_3 \leftrightarrow H^+ + HCO_3^-.$$

CO_2 dissolved in plasma is in equilibrium with CO_2 in the lung alveoli (expressed as a partial pressure [P_{CO_2}]). Thus, an equilibrium exists between alveolar P_{CO_2} and the various forms of CO_2 present in the plasma, as expressed by the following formula:

$$P_{CO_2} \leftrightarrow CO_2 + H_2O \leftrightarrow H_2CO_3 \leftrightarrow H + HCO_3^-.$$

Don't hold your breath!

A change in the rate or depth of respirations can alter the CO_2 content of alveolar air and the alveolar P_{CO_2}. A change in alveolar P_{CO_2} produces a corresponding change in the amount of H_2CO_3 formed by dissolved CO_2. In turn, these changes stimulate the respiratory center to modify respiratory rate and depth.

An increase in alveolar P_{CO_2} raises the blood concentration of CO_2 and H_2CO_3. This, in turn, stimulates the respiratory center to increase respiratory rate and depth. As a result, alveolar P_{CO_2} decreases, which leads to a corresponding drop in the H_2CO_3 and CO_2 concentrations in blood. (See *How respiratory mechanisms affect blood pH.*)

A decrease in respiratory rate and depth has the reverse effect; it raises alveolar P_{CO_2} which, in turn, triggers an increase in the blood's CO_2 and H_2CO_3 concentrations.

Kidneys

In addition to excreting various acid waste products, the kidneys help manage acid-base balance by regulating the blood's HCO_3^- concentration. They do so by permitting HCO_3^- reabsorption from tubular filtrate and by forming additional HCO_3^- to replace that used in buffering acids.

Renal tubular ion secretion

Recovery and formation of HCO_3^- in the kidneys depend on H ion secretion by the renal tubules in exchange for sodium (Na) ions. Na ions are then simultaneously reabsorbed into the circulation from the tubular filtrate.

Now I get it!

How respiratory mechanisms affect blood pH

A rise in the carbon dioxide (CO_2) content of arterial blood or a decrease in blood pH stimulates the respiratory center, causing *hyperventilation*. As a result, less CO_2 and, therefore, less carbonic acid and fewer hydrogen ions remain in the blood. Consequently, blood pH increases, possibly reaching a normal level.

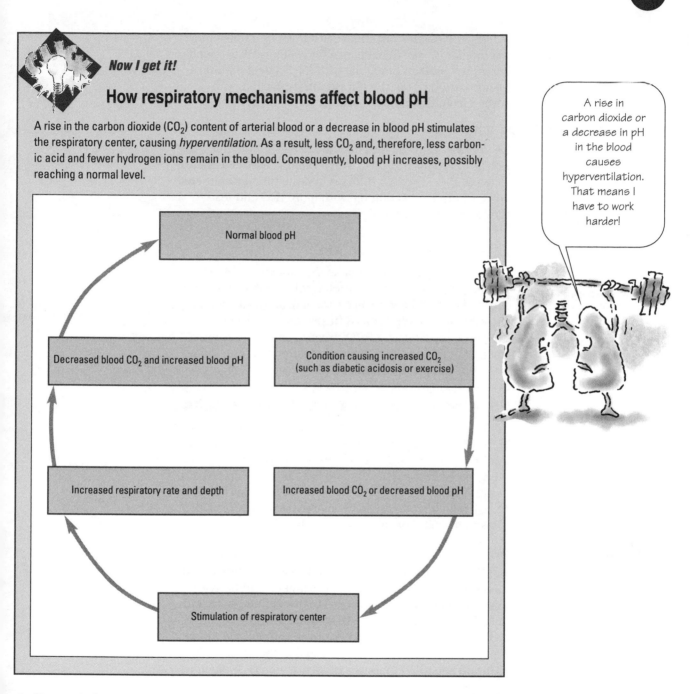

A rise in carbon dioxide or a decrease in pH in the blood causes hyperventilation. That means I have to work harder!

Influential enzyme

The enzyme *carbonic anhydrase* influences tubular epithelial cells to form H_2CO_3 from CO_2 and H_2O. H_2CO_3

quickly dissociates into H and HCO_3^- ions. H ions enter the tubular filtrate in exchange for Na ions; HCO_3^- ions enter the bloodstream along with the Na ions that have been absorbed from the filtrate. HCO_3^- is then reabsorbed from the tubular filtrate.

Ions hanging out together

Each H ion secreted into the tubular filtrate joins with an HCO_3^- ion to form H_2CO_3, which rapidly dissociates into CO_2 and H_2O. The CO_2 diffuses into the tubular epithelial cells, where it can combine with more H_2O and lead to the formation of more H_2CO_3.

Bicarbonate reabsorption

The remaining H_2O molecule in the tubular filtrate is eliminated in the urine. As each H ion enters the tubular filtrate to combine with an HCO_3^- ion, an HCO_3^- ion in the tubular epithelial cells diffuses into the circulation. This process is termed HCO_3^- reabsorption. (However, the HCO_3^- ion that enters the circulation isn't the same one as in the tubular filtrate.)

Formation of ammonia and phosphate salts

To form more HCO_3^-, the kidneys must secrete additional H ions in exchange for Na ions. For the renal tubules to continue secreting H ions, the excess ions must combine with other substances in the filtrate and be excreted. Excess H ions in the filtrate may combine with *ammonia* (NH_3), which is produced by the renal tubules, or with phosphate salts present in the tubular filtrate.

More ions on the move

NH_3 forms in the tubular epithelial cells by removal of the amino groups from *glutamine* (an amino acid derivative) and from amino acids delivered to the tubular epithelial cells from the circulation. After diffusing into the filtrate, NH_3 joins with the secreted H ions, forming ammonium ions (NH_4^+). These ions are excreted in the urine with chloride and other anions; each secreted NH_3 molecule eliminates one H ion in the filtrate.

At the same time, Na ions that have been absorbed from the filtrate and exchanged for H ions enter the circulation, as does the HCO_3^- formed in the tubular epithelial cells. Some secreted H ions combine with Na_2HPO_4, a *disodium phosphate salt* in the tubular filtrate. Each of the secreted H ions that joins with the disodium salt changes to the monosodium salt NaH_2PO_4. The Na ion released in this reaction is absorbed into the circulation along with a newly formed HCO_3^- ion.

Factors affecting bicarbonate formation

The rate of HCO_3^- formation by renal tubular epithelial cells is affected by two factors:
- the amount of dissolved CO_2 in the plasma
- the potassium (K) content of the tubular cells.

If the plasma CO_2 level rises, renal tubular cells form more HCO_3^-. Increased plasma CO_2 encourages greater H_2CO_3 formation by the renal tubular cells.

Chain reaction

Partial dissociation of H_2CO_3 results in more H ions for excretion into the tubular filtrate and additional HCO_3^- ions for entry into the circulation. This, in turn, increases the plasma HCO_3^- level and reduces the plasma level of dissolved CO_2 toward normal. If the plasma CO_2 level decreases, renal tubular cells form less H_2CO_3.

Because fewer H ions are formed and excreted, fewer HCO_3^- ions enter the circulation. The plasma HCO_3^- level then falls accordingly.

Special K

The K content of renal tubular cells also helps regulate plasma HCO_3^- concentration by affecting the rate at which the renal tubules secrete H ions. Tubular cell K content and H ion secretion are interrelated; K and H ions are secreted at rates that vary inversely. H ion secretion increases if tubular secretion of K ions falls; H ion secretion declines if tubular secretion of K ions increases.

For each H ion secreted into the tubular filtrate, an additional HCO_3^- ion enters the blood plasma. Consequently, increased tubular secretion of H ions leads to a rise in the plasma HCO_3^- content.

Depletion of body K causes more HCO_3^- to enter the circulation; the plasma HCO_3^- level then rises above normal. When the body contains excess K, the tubules excrete more K. As a result, fewer H ions are secreted, less HCO_3^- forms, and the plasma HCO_3^- concentration decreases.

Potassium secretion by tubular epithelial cells decreases and hydrogen ion secretion rises in patients with potassium depletion from vomiting or diarrhea.

Quick quiz

1. A solution with a pH of less than 7 is considered:
    A. acidic.
    B. alkaline.
    C. solute.
    D. hypotonic.

Answer: A. A solution with a pH of less than 7 contains more H ions than OH^- ions and is considered acidic.

2. The body compensates for chronic respiratory alkalosis by developing:
    A. metabolic alkalosis.
    B. respiratory acidosis.
    C. metabolic acidosis.
    D. a phosphate buffer system.

Answer: C. The body compensates for chronic respiratory alkalosis by developing metabolic acidosis.

3. The two factors that affect the rate of HCO_3^- formation by renal tubular epithelial cells are:
    A. amount of aldosterone in the system and urine production.
    B. amount of dissolved CO_2 in the plasma and the K content of the tubular cells.
    C. amount of dissolved K in the plasma and the CO_2 content of the tubular cells.
    D. amount of ammonia produced by the renal tubules and the phosphate salts present in the tubular filtrate.

Answer: B. The rate of HCO_3^- formation by renal tubular epithelial cells is affected by the amount of dissolved CO_2 in the plasma and the K content of tubular cells.

Scoring

☆☆☆ If you answered all three questions correctly, give yourself a pat on the back! You have all your knowledge in the proper balance.

☆☆ If you answered two questions correctly, good for you! You're benefiting from all the right buffer systems.

☆ If you answered only one question correctly, check out this chapter again. It may take time to find your equilibrium.

Reproductive system

Just the facts

In this chapter, you'll learn:

♦ anatomic structure and functions of the male and female reproductive systems

♦ male hormone production and its effects on sexual development

♦ female hormone production and its effects on menstruation

♦ anatomic structure and functions of the female breast.

A look at the reproductive systems

Anatomically, the main distinction between the male and female is the presence of conspicuous external genitalia in the male versus the internal (within the pelvic cavity) location of the major reproductive organs in the female.

Here's the main difference — males have major external genitalia...

...but most female reproductive organs are inside the pelvic cavity.

Male reproductive system

The male reproductive system consists of the organs that produce, transfer, and introduce mature sperm into the female reproductive tract, where fertilization occurs. (See *Structures of the male reproductive system.*)

Extra work

In addition to forming male sex cells (spermatogenesis), the male reproductive system plays a role in the secretion of male sex hormones.

Zoom in

Structures of the male reproductive system

The male reproductive system consists of the penis, the scrotum and its contents, the prostate gland, and the inguinal structures. These structures are illustrated below.

Penis

The organ of copulation, the *penis* deposits sperm in the female reproductive tract and acts as the terminal duct for the urinary tract. The penis also serves as the conduit for urine elimination. It consists of an attached root, a free shaft, and an enlarged tip.

From the inside...

Internally, the cylinder-shaped penile shaft consists of three columns of *erectile tissue* bound together by *heavy fibrous tissue*. Two *corpora cavernosa* form the major part of the penis. On the underside, the *corpus spongiosum* encases the urethra. The enlarged proximal end of the urethra forms the bulb of the penis.

The *glans penis*, at the distal end of the shaft, is a cone-shaped structure formed from the corpus spongiosum. Its lateral margin forms a ridge of tissue known as the *corona*. The glans penis is highly sensitive to sexual stimulation.

...out

Thin, loose skin covers the penile shaft. The *urethral meatus* opens through the glans to allow urination and ejaculation.

In a different vein

The penis receives blood through the *internal pudendal artery*. Blood then flows into the corpora cavernosa through the penile artery. Venous blood returns through the *internal iliac vein* to the *vena cava*.

Scrotum

The penis meets the *scrotum*, or scrotal sac, at the penoscrotal junction. Located posterior to the penis and anterior to the anus, the scrotum is an extra-abdominal pouch that consists of a thin layer of skin overlying a tighter, musclelike layer. This musclelike layer overlies the tunica vaginalis, a serous membrane that covers the internal scrotal cavity.

Canals and rings

Internally, a *septum* divides the scrotum into two sacs, which each contain a *testis*, an *epididymis*, and a *sper-*

matic cord. The spermatic cord is a connective tissue sheath that encases autonomic nerve fibers, blood vessels, lymph vessels, and the *vas deferens* (also called the *ductus deferens*).

The spermatic cord travels from the testis through the inguinal canal, exiting the scrotum through the external inguinal ring and entering the abdominal cavity through the internal inguinal ring. The inguinal canal lies between the two rings.

Loads of nodes

Lymph nodes from the penis, scrotal surface, and anus drain into the *inguinal* lymph nodes. Lymph nodes from the testes drain into the lateral aortic and pre-aortic lymph nodes in the abdomen.

Testes

The testes are enveloped in two layers of connective tissue: the *tunica vaginalis* (outer layer) and the *tunica albuginea* (inner layer). Extensions of the tunica albuginea separate each testis into lobules. Each lobule contains one to four *seminiferous tubules*, small tubes in which spermatogenesis takes place.

Climate control

Spermatozoa development requires a temperature lower than that of the rest of the body. The *dartos muscle*, a smooth muscle in the superficial fascia, causes scrotal skin to wrinkle, which helps to regulate temperature. The *cremaster muscle*, rising from the internal oblique muscle, helps to govern temperature by elevating the testes.

An important function of the scrotum is to keep the testes cooler than the rest of the body.

Duct system

The male reproductive *duct system*, consisting of the epididymis, vas deferens, and urethra, conveys sperm from the testes to the ejaculatory ducts near the bladder.

Swimmer storage

The *epididymis* is a coiled tube located superior to and along the posterior border of the testis. During ejaculation, smooth muscle in the epididymis contracts, ejecting spermatozoa into the vas deferens.

Descending and merging

The *vas deferens* leads from the testes to the abdominal cavity, where it extends upward through the *inguinal canal*, arches over the urethra, and descends behind the bladder. Its enlarged portion, called the *ampulla*, merges with the duct of the seminal vesicle to form the short ejaculatory duct. After passing through the prostate gland, the vas deferens joins with the urethra.

Tubular exit

A small tube leading from the floor of the bladder to the exterior, the *urethra* consists of three parts:
• *prostatic urethra* (surrounded by the prostate gland), which drains the bladder
• *membranous urethra*, which passes through the urogenital diaphragm
• *spongy urethra*, which makes up about 75% of the entire urethra.

During ejaculation, smooth muscle in the epididymis contracts, sending spermatozoa into the vas deferens.

Accessory reproductive glands

The accessory reproductive glands, which produce most of the semen, include the *seminal vesicles, bulbourethral glands (Cowper's glands)*, and the *prostate gland*. The seminal vesicles are paired sacs at the base of the bladder. The bulbourethral glands, also paired, are located inferior to the prostate.

Size of a walnut

The walnut-sized prostate gland lies under the bladder and surrounds the urethra. It consists of three lobes: the left and right lateral lobes and the median lobe.

Improving the odds

The prostate continuously secretes prostatic fluid, a thin, milky, alkaline fluid. During sexual activity, prostatic fluid adds volume to the semen. The fluid enhances sperm motility and may improve the odds for conception by neutralizing the acidity of the man's urethra and the woman's vagina.

Slightly alkaline

Semen is a viscous, white secretion with a slightly alkaline pH (7.8 to 8); it consists of spermatozoa and accessory gland secretions. The seminal vesicles produce rough-ly 60% of the fluid portion of the semen, while the prostate gland produces about 30%. A viscid fluid secret-ed by the bulbourethral glands also becomes part of the semen.

Spermatogenesis

Sperm formation, or *spermatogenesis*, begins when a male reaches *puberty* and normally continues throughout life.

Memory jogger

To remem-ber the meaning of sper-matogenesis, keep in mind that *genesis* means "beginning" or "new." Therefore, *spermatogenesis* means beginning of new sperm.

Divide and conquer

Spermatogenesis occurs in four stages:

☝ In the first stage, the primary germinal epithelial cells, called *spermatogonia*, grow and develop into pri-mary *spermatocytes*. Both spermatogonia and primary spermatocytes contain 46 chromosomes, consisting of 44 *autosomes* and the two sex chromosomes, X and Y.

✌ Next, primary spermatocytes divide to form sec-ondary spermatocytes. No new chromosomes are formed in this stage; the pairs only divide. Each secondary sper-matocyte contains half the number of autosomes, 22. One secondary spermatocyte contains an X chromosome; the other, a Y chromosome.

🤟 In the third stage, each secondary spermatocyte di-vides again to form *spermatids* (also called *spermato-blasts*).

🖐 Finally, the spermatids undergo a series of structural changes that transform them into mature *spermatozoa*, or sperm. Each spermatozoa has a head, neck, body, and tail. The head contains the *nucleus*; the tail, a large amount of *adenosine triphosphate*, which provides ener-gy for sperm *motility*.

I'm newly mature and ready for emission.

Queuing up

Newly mature sperm pass from the seminiferous tubules through the *vasa recta* into the epididymis. Only a small number of sperm can be stored in the epididymis. Most of them move into the vas deferens, where they're stored until sexu-al stimulation triggers emission.

Keeps for weeks

Sperm cells retain their potency in storage for many weeks. After ejaculation, sperm can survive for up to 4 days in the female reproductive tract.

Number and motility affect fertility. A low sperm count (less than 20 million per milliliter of ejaculated semen) may cause infertility.

Hormonal control and sexual development

Androgens (male sex hormones) are produced in the testes and the adrenal glands. They're responsible for the development of male sex organs and secondary sex characteristics. Major androgens include:
• testosterone
• luteinizing hormone (LH)
• follicle-stimulating hormone (FSH).

The captain of the team

Leydig's cells, located in the testes between the seminiferous tubules, secrete *testosterone*, the most significant male sex hormone. Testosterone is responsible for the development and maintenance of male sex organs and secondary sex characteristics, such as facial hair and vocal cord thickness. Testosterone is also required for spermatogenesis.

Calling the plays

Testosterone secretion begins approximately 2 months after conception, when the release of chorionic gonadotropins from the placenta stimulates Leydig's cells in the male fetus. The presence of testosterone directly affects sexual differentiation in the fetus. With testosterone, fetal genitalia develop into a penis, scrotum, and testes; without testosterone, genitalia develop into a clitoris, vagina, and other female organs.

During the last 2 months of gestation, testosterone normally causes the testes to descend into the scrotum. If the testes don't descend after birth, exogenous testosterone may correct the problem.

Other key players

Other hormones also affect male sexuality. Two of these, *LH* (also called *interstitial cell-stimulating hormone*) and *FSH*, directly affect secretion of testosterone.

Time to grow

During early childhood, a boy doesn't secrete gonadotropins and thus has little circulating testosterone. Secretion of gonadotropins from the pituitary gland, which usually occurs between ages 11 and 14, marks the onset of *puberty*. These pituitary gonadotropins stimulate testis functioning as well as testosterone secretion.

No gonadotropins yet.

From boy to man

During puberty, the penis and testes enlarge and the male reaches full adult sexual and reproductive capability. Puberty also marks the development of male secondary sexual characteristics: distinct body hair distribution, skin changes (such as increased secretion by sweat and sebaceous glands), deepening of the voice (from laryngeal enlargement), increased musculoskeletal development, and other intracellular and extracellular changes.

Reaching the plateau

After a male achieves full physical maturity, usually by age 20, sexual and reproductive function remain fairly consistent throughout life. (See *Male reproductive changes with aging*.)

Senior moment

Male reproductive changes with aging

Physiologic changes in older men include reduced testosterone production which, in turn, may cause decreased libido. A reduced testosterone level also causes the testes to atrophy and soften and decreases sperm production by 48% to 69% between ages 60 and 80.

Normally, the prostate gland enlarges with age and its secretions diminish. Seminal fluid also decreases in volume and becomes less viscous.

Sexual changes
During intercourse, older men experience slower and weaker physiologic reactions. However, these changes don't necessarily lessen sexual satisfaction.

Female reproductive system

Unlike the male reproductive system, the female system is largely internal, housed within the pelvic cavity.

External genitalia

The vulva contains the external female genitalia, those visible on inspection, including the *mons pubis, labia majora, labia minora, clitoris*, and adjacent structures. (See *Structures of the female reproductive system*, pages 278 and 279.)

At the bottom

The *mons pubis* is a rounded cushion of fatty and connective tissue covered by skin and coarse, curly hair in a triangular pattern over the symphysis pubis (the joint formed by the union of the pubic bones anteriorly).

Major league

The *labia majora* are two raised folds of adipose and connective tissue that border the vulva on either side, extending from the mons pubis to the perineum. After *menarche* (onset of menses), the outer surface of the labia is covered with pubic hair. The inner surface is pink and moist.

Minor...

The *labia minora* are two moist folds of mucosal tissue, dark pink to red in color, that lie within and alongside the labia majora. Each upper section divides into an upper and lower lamella. The two upper lamellae join to form the *prepuce*, a hoodlike covering over the clitoris. The two lower lamellae form the *frenulum*, the posterior portion of the clitoris.

The lower labial sections taper down and back from the clitoris to the perineum, where they join to form the *fourchette*, a thin tissue fold along the anterior edge of the perineum.

...in name only

The labia minora contain sebaceous glands, which secrete a lubricant that also acts as a bactericide. Like the labia majora, they're rich in blood vessels and nerve end-

> The labia are highly vascular and have many nerve endings — making them sensitive to pain, pressure, touch, sexual stimulation, and temperature extremes.

Zoom in

Structures of the female reproductive system

The female reproductive system includes the vagina, cervix, uterus, fallopian tubes, ovaries, and other structures. These structures are illustrated here.

View of external genitalia in lithotomy position

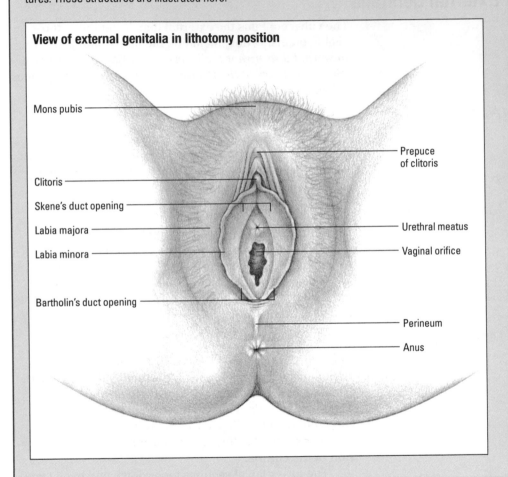

Mons pubis

Prepuce
of clitoris

Clitoris

Skene's duct opening

Labia majora

Urethral meatus

Labia minora

Vaginal orifice

Bartholin's duct opening

Perineum

Anus

ings, which makes them highly responsive to stimulation.
They swell in response to sexual stimulation, a reaction
that triggers other changes that prepare the genitalia for
coitus.

Small but sensitive

The *clitoris* is the small, protuberant organ just beneath
the arch of the mons pubis. It contains erectile tissue, ve-

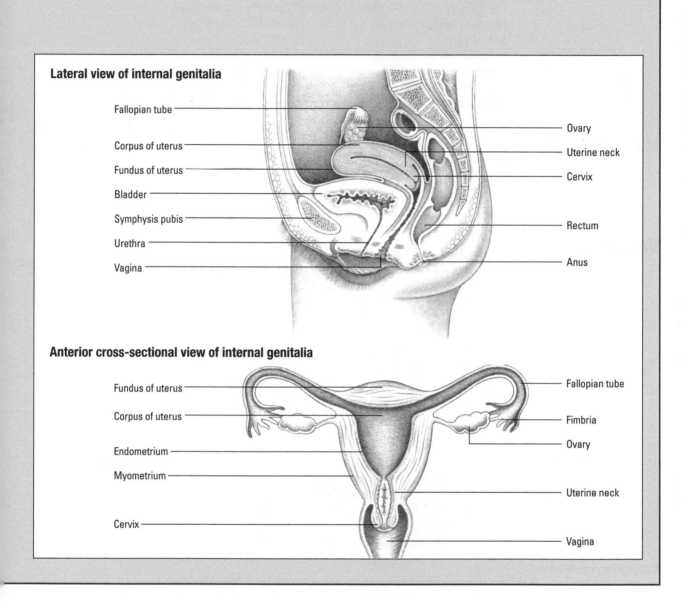

Lateral view of internal genitalia

- Fallopian tube
- Corpus of uterus
- Fundus of uterus
- Bladder
- Symphysis pubis
- Urethra
- Vagina
- Ovary
- Uterine neck
- Cervix
- Rectum
- Anus

Anterior cross-sectional view of internal genitalia

- Fundus of uterus
- Corpus of uterus
- Endometrium
- Myometrium
- Cervix
- Fallopian tube
- Fimbria
- Ovary
- Uterine neck
- Vagina

nous cavernous spaces, and specialized sensory corpuscles, which are stimulated during sexual activity.

Mucho mucus

The *vestibule* is an oval area bounded anteriorly by the clitoris, laterally by the labia minora, and posteriorly by the fourchette. The mucus-producing *Skene's glands* are found on both sides of the urethral opening. Openings of the two mucus-producing *Bartholin's glands* are located laterally and posteriorly on either side of the inner vaginal orifice.

The *urethral meatus* is the slitlike opening below the clitoris through which urine leaves the body. In the center of the vestibule is the *vaginal orifice.* It may be completely or partially covered by the *hymen,* a tissue membrane.

Not too simple

Located between the lower vagina and the anal canal, the *perineum* is a complex structure of muscles, blood vessels, fasciae, nerves, and lymphatics.

Vagina

The female internal genitalia, beginning with the vagina, are specialized organs; their main function is reproduction.

Three layers...

The *vagina,* a highly elastic muscular tube, is located between the urethra and the rectum. The vaginal wall has three tissue layers: epithelial tissue, loose connective tissue, and muscle tissue. The *uterine cervix* connects the uterus to the vaginal vault. Four *fornices,* recesses in the vaginal wall, surround the cervix.

...three functions

The vagina has three main functions:
• accommodating the penis during coitus
• channeling blood discharged from the uterus during menstruation
• serving as the birth canal during childbirth.

Supplied separately

The upper, middle, and lower vaginal sections have separate blood supplies. Branches of the uterine arteries supply blood to the upper vagina, the *inferior vesical arteries* supply blood to the middle vagina, and the hemorrhoidal and *internal pudendal arteries* feed into the lower vagina.

Blood returns through a vast venous *plexus* to the hemorrhoidal, pudendal, and uterine veins and then to the *hypogastric* veins. This plexus merges with the *vertebral venous plexus.*

Cervix

The cervix projects into the upper portion of the vagina. The lower cervical opening is the *external os;* the upper opening is the *internal os.*

Permanent alterations

Childbirth permanently alters the cervix. In a female who hasn't delivered a child, the external os is a round opening about 3 mm in diameter; after the first childbirth, it becomes a small transverse slit with irregular edges.

Uterus

The *uterus* is a small, firm, pear-shaped, muscular organ that's situated between the bladder and rectum. It typically lies at nearly a 90-degree angle to the vagina. The mucous membrane lining of the uterus is called the *endometrium,* and the muscular layer of the uterus is called the *myometrium.*

Fundamental fundus

During pregnancy, the elastic, upper portion of the uterus, called the *fundus,* accommodates most of the growing fetus until term. The uterine neck joins the fundus to the cervix, the part of the uterus that extends into the vagina. The fundus and neck make up the *corpus,* the main uterine body.

Fallopian tubes

Two *fallopian tubes* attach to the uterus at the upper angles of the fundus. These narrow cylinders of muscle fibers are the site of fertilization.

Riding the wave

The curved portion of the fallopian tube, called the *ampulla,* ends in the funnel-shaped *infundibulum.* Fingerlike projections in the infundibulum, called *fimbriae,* move in waves that sweep the mature ovum from the ovary into the fallopian tube.

Fingerlike projections called fimbriae move in waves, sweeping the ovum from the ovary to the fallopian tube.

Ovaries

The *ovaries* are located on either side of the uterus. The size, shape, and position of the ovaries vary with age. Round, smooth, and pink at birth, they grow larger, flatten, and turn grayish by puberty. During the childbearing years, they take on an almond shape and a rough, pitted surface; after menopause, they shrink and turn white.

500,000 follicles

The ovaries' main function is to produce mature ova. At birth, each ovary contains approximately 500,000 *graafian follicles*. During the childbearing years, one graafian follicle produces a mature ovum during the first half of each menstrual cycle. As the ovum matures, the follicle ruptures and the ovum is swept into the fallopian tube.

The ovaries also produce estrogen, progesterone, and a small amount of androgens.

Mammary glands

The mammary glands, which are located in the breasts, are specialized accessory glands that secrete milk. Although present in both sexes, they typically function only in the female.

Lobes, ducts, and drainage

Each mammary gland contains 15 to 25 lobes separated by fibrous connective tissue and fat. Within the lobes are clustered acini — tiny, saclike duct terminals that secrete milk during lactation.

The ducts draining the lobules converge to form excretory (*lactiferous*) ducts and sinuses (*ampullae*), which store milk during lactation. These ducts drain onto the nipple surface through 15 to 20 openings. (See *The female breast*.)

Males and females have mammary glands — but they function only in the female.

Hormonal function and the menstrual cycle

Like the male body, the female body changes with age in response to hormonal control. (See *Events in the female reproductive cycle*, pages 284 and 285.) When a female reaches the age of menstruation, the hypothalamus, ovaries, and pituitary gland secrete hormones — *estro-*

(Text continues on page 286.)

Zoom in

The female breast

The breasts are located on either side of the anterior chest wall over the greater pectoral and the anterior serratus muscles. Within the areola, the pigmented area in the center of the breast, lies the nipple. Erectile tissue in the nipple responds to cold, friction, and sexual stimulation.

Support and separate

Each breast is composed of glandular, fibrous, and adipose tissue. Glandular tissue contains 15 to 20 lobes made up of clustered *acini*, tiny saclike duct terminals that secrete milk. Fibrous *Cooper's ligaments* support the breasts; *adipose tissue* surrounds each breast.

Produce and drain

Acini draw the ingredients needed to produce milk from the blood in surrounding capillaries.

Sebaceous glands on the areolar surface, called *Montgomery's tubercles*, produce *sebum*, which lubricates the areolae and nipples during breast-feeding.

Lateral cross section

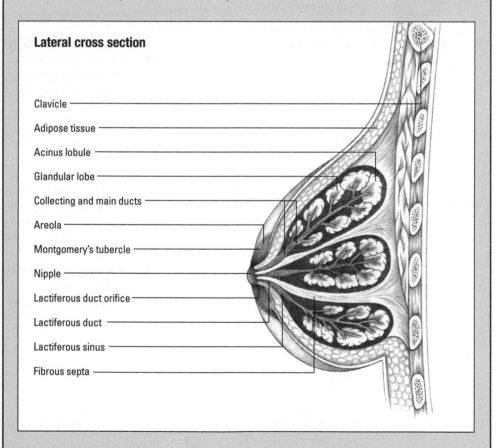

Clavicle

Adipose tissue

Acinus lobule

Glandular lobe

Collecting and main ducts

Areola

Montgomery's tubercle

Nipple

Lactiferous duct orifice

Lactiferous duct

Lactiferous sinus

Fibrous septa

There are three major types of changes during the reproductive cycle: ovulatory, hormonal, and endometrial.

Now I get it!

Events in the female reproductive cycle

The female reproductive cycle usually lasts 28 days. During this cycle, three major types of changes occur simultaneously: ovulatory, hormonal, and endometrial (involving the lining [endometrium] of the uterus).

Ovulatory

- Ovulatory changes begin on the 1st day of the menstrual cycle.
- As the cycle begins, low estrogen and progesterone levels in the bloodstream stimulate the hypothalamus to secrete gonadotropin-stimulating hormone (Gn-RH). In turn, Gn-RH stimulates the anterior pituitary gland to secrete follicle-stimulating hormone (FSH) and luteinizing hormone (LH).
- Follicle development within the ovary (in the follicular phase) is spurred by increased levels of FSH and, to a lesser extent, LH.
- When the follicle matures, a spike in the LH level occurs, causing the follicle to rupture and release the ovum, thus initiating ovulation.
- After ovulation (in the luteal phase), the collapsed follicle forms the corpus luteum, which (if fertilization doesn't occur) degenerates.

Hormonal

- During the follicular phase of the ovarian cycle, the increasing FSH and LH levels that stimulate follicle growth also stimulate increased secretion of estrogen.
- Estrogen secretion peaks just before ovulation. This peak sets in motion the spike in LH levels, which causes ovulation.
- After ovulation, estrogen levels decline rapidly. In the luteal phase of the ovarian cycle, the corpus luteum is formed and beings to release progesterone and estrogen.
- As the corpus luteum degenerates, levels of both of these ovarian hormones decline.

Endometrial

- The endometrium is receptive to implantation of an embryo for only a short time in the reproductive cycle. Thus, it's no accident that the endometrium is most receptive about 7 days after the initiation of ovulation — just in time to receive a fertilized ovum.
- In the first 5 days of the reproductive cycle, the endometrium sheds its functional layer, leaving the basal layer (the deepest layer) intact. Menstrual flow consists of this detached layer and accompanying blood from the detachment process.
- The endometrium begins regenerating its functional layer at about day 6 (the proliferative phase), spurred by rising estrogen levels.
- After ovulation (about day 14), increased progesterone secretion stimulates conversion of the functional layer into a secretory mucosa (secretory phase), which is more receptive to implantation of the fertilized ovum.
- If implantation doesn't occur, the corpus luteum degenerates, progesterone levels drop, and the endometrium again sheds its functional layer.

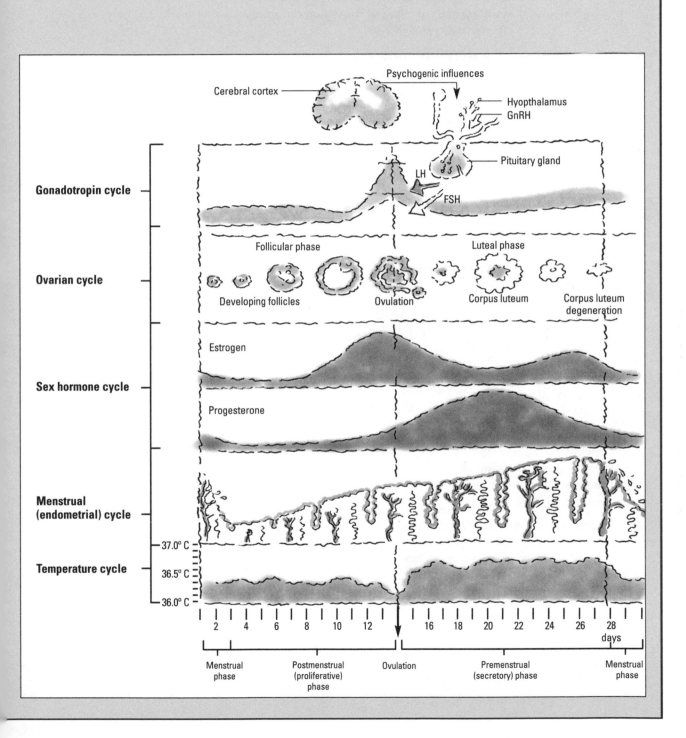

gen, progesterone, FSH, and *LH* — that affect the buildup and shedding of the endometrium during the menstrual cycle.

A sometimes shocking development

During adolescence, the release of hormones causes a rapid increase in physical growth and spurs the development of secondary sex characteristics. This growth spurt begins at approximately age 11 and continues until early adolescence, or about 3 years later.

Senior moment

Female reproductive changes with aging

Declining estrogen and progesterone levels cause numerous physical changes in aging women. Because women's breasts and internal and external reproductive structures are estrogen-dependent, aging takes a more conspicuous toll on women than on men. As estrogen levels decrease and menopause approaches, usually at about age 50, changes affect most parts of the female reproductive system. Significant emotional changes also take place during the transition from childbearing years to infertility.

Ovaries
Ovulation usually stops 1 to 2 years before menopause. As the ovaries reach the end of their productive cycle, they become unresponsive to gonadotropic stimulation. With aging, the ovaries atrophy and become thicker and smaller.

Vulva
The vulva also atrophies with age. Vulval tissue shrinks, exposing the sensitive area around the urethra and vagina to abrasions and irritations—from undergarments, for example. The introitus also constricts, tissues lose their elasticity, and the epidermis thins from 20 layers to about 5. Other changes include pubic hair loss and flattening of the labia majora.

Vagina
Atrophy causes the vagina to shorten and the mucous lining to become thin, dry, less elastic, and pale from decreased vascularity. In this state, the vaginal mucosa is highly susceptible to abrasion. In addition, the pH of vaginal secretions increases,

making the vaginal environment more alkaline. The type of flora in it also changes, increasing older women's risk of vaginal infections.

Uterus
After menopause, the uterus shrinks rapidly to half its premenstrual weight. It continues to shrink until the organ reaches approximately one-fourth its premenstrual size. The cervix atrophies and no longer produces mucus for lubrication, and the endometrium and myometrium become thinner.

Breasts
In the breasts, glandular, supporting, and fatty tissues atrophy. As Cooper's ligaments lose their elasticity, the breasts become pendulous. The nipples decrease in size and become flat, and the inframammary ridges become more pronounced.

Pelvic support structures
Relaxation of the pelvic support commonly occurs in postreproductive women. Initial relaxation usually occurs during labor and delivery, but clinical effects commonly go unnoticed until the process accelerates with menopausal estrogen depletion and loss of connective tissue elasticity and tone. Signs and symptoms include pressure and pulling sensations in the area above the inguinal ligaments, lower backaches, a feeling of pelvic heaviness, and difficulty in rising from a sitting position. Urinary stress incontinence may also become a problem if urethrovesical ligaments weaken.

Menarche, the onset of menstruation, generally occurs after this growth spurt, usually between ages 11 and 14. Irregularity of the menstrual cycle is common during this time because of failure to ovulate. With menarche, the uterine body flexes on the cervix and the ovaries are situated in the pelvic cavity.

> The menstrual cycle may range from 22 to 34 days, although the typical cycle lasts 28 days.

A monthly thing

The menstrual cycle is a complex process that involves the reproductive and endocrine systems. The cycle averages 28 days in length.

Supply exhausted

Cessation of menses usually occurs between ages 40 and 55. Although the pituitary gland still releases FSH and LH, the body has exhausted the supply of ovarian follicles that respond to these hormones, and menstruation no longer occurs.

A farewell to menses

A woman is considered to have reached menopause after menses are absent for 1 year. Before menopause, a woman experiences several transitional years (called the *climacteric years*), during which several physiologic changes that lead to menopause occur. (See *Female reproductive changes with aging.*)

Quick quiz

1. Spermatogenesis is the:
   A. growth and development of sperm into primary spermatocytes.
   B. division of spermatocytes into secondary spermatocytes.
   C. passage of sperm into the epididymis.
   D. entire process of sperm formation.

Answer: D. Spermatogenesis refers to the entire process of sperm formation, from the development of primary spermatocytes to the formation of fully functional spermatozoa.

2. The primary function of the scrotum is to:
    A.   provide storage for newly developed sperm.
    B.   maintain a cool temperature for the testes.
    C.   deposit sperm in the female reproductive tract.
    D.   secrete prostatic fluid.

Answer: B. The scrotum maintains a cool temperature for the testes, which is necessary for spermatozoa formation.

3. The main function of the ovaries is to:
    A.   secrete hormones that affect the buildup and shedding of the endometrium during the menstrual cycle.
    B.   accommodate a growing fetus during pregnancy.
    C.   produce mature ova.
    D.   serve as the site of fertilization.

Answer: C. The main function of the ovaries is to produce mature ova.

4. The corpus luteum forms and degenerates in which phase of the female reproductive cycle?
    A.   Luteal
    B.   Follicular
    C.   Proliferative
    D.   Secretory

Answer: A. The corpus luteum forms and degenerates in the luteal phase of the ovarian cycle.

5. Four hormones involved in the menstrual cycle are:
    A.   LH, progesterone, estrogen, and testosterone.
    B.   estrogen, FSH, LH, and androgens.
    C.   estrogen, progesterone, LH, and FSH.
    D.   gonadotropin-stimulating hormone, estrogen, progesterone, and testosterone.

Answer: C. The four hormones involved in the menstrual cycle are estrogen, progesterone, LH, and FSH.

Scoring

☆☆☆ If you answered all five questions correctly, congrats! You've hit a growth spurt in your knowledge.

☆☆ If you answered four questions correctly, good for you! You have a firm grasp of this complicated system.

☆ If you answered fewer than four questions correctly, keep trying! Like the reproductive system, your knowledge may just need some time to develop.

Reproduction and lactation

Just the facts

In this chapter, you'll learn:
♦ the process of fertilization
♦ embryo and fetus development
♦ stages of labor
♦ the role of hormones in lactation.

Fertilization

Creation of a new human being begins with *fertilization*, the union of a *spermatozoon* and an *ovum* to form a single cell. After fertilization occurs, dramatic changes begin inside a woman's body. The cells of the fertilized ovum begin dividing as the ovum travels to the *uterine cavity*, where it implants in the uterine lining. (See *How fertilization occurs*, page 290.)

One in a million

For fertilization to take place, however, a spermatozoon must first reach the ovum. Although a single ejaculation deposits several hundred-million spermatozoa, many are destroyed by acidic vaginal secretions. The only spermatozoa that survive are those that enter the *cervical canal*, where they're protected by *cervical mucus*.

Timing is everything

The ability of spermatozoa to penetrate the cervical mucus depends on the phase of the menstrual cycle at the time of transit.

Early in the cycle, estrogen and progesterone levels cause the mucus to thicken, making it more difficult for

Now I get it!

How fertilization occurs

Fertilization begins when a spermatozoon is activated upon contact with the ovum. Here's what happens.

The spermatozoon, which has a covering called the *acrosome,* approaches the ovum.

Ovum

Acrosome

Spermatozoon

The acrosome develops small perforations through which it releases enzymes necessary for the sperm to penetrate the protective layers of the ovum before fertilization.

Enzymes released

Dispersed granulosa cells

The spermatozoon then penetrates the zona pellucida (the inner membrane of the ovum). This triggers the ovum's second meiotic division (following meiosis), making the zona pellucida impenetrable to other spermatozoa.

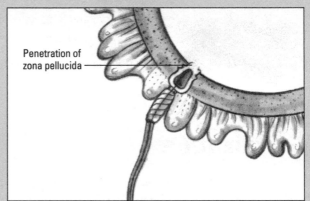

Penetration of zona pellucida

After the spermatozoon penetrates the ovum, its nucleus is released into the ovum, its tail degenerates, and its head enlarges and fuses with the ovum's nucleus. This fusion provides the fertilized ovum, called a *zygote,* with 46 chromosomes.

Spermatozoon nucleus released into the ovum

spermatozoa to pass through the cervix. During midcycle, however, when the mucus is relatively thin, spermatozoa can pass readily through the cervix. Later in the cycle, the cervical mucus thickens again, hindering spermatozoa passage.

Help along the way

Spermatozoa travel through the female reproductive tract at a rate of several millimeters per hour by means of whiplike movements of the tail, known as *flagellar movements*.

After spermatozoa pass through the cervical mucus, however, the female reproductive system "assists" them on their journey with rhythmic contractions of the uterus that help them penetrate the fallopian tubes. Spermatozoa are typically viable (able to fertilize the ovum) for up to 2 days after ejaculation; however, they can survive in the reproductive tract for up to 4 days.

A zygote is "born"

Before a spermatozoon can penetrate the ovum, it must disperse the *granulosa* cells (outer protective cells) and penetrate the *zona pellucida* — the thick, transparent layer surrounding the incompletely developed ovum. Enzymes in the *acrosome* (head cap) of the spermatozoon permit this penetration. After penetration, the ovum completes its second meiotic division, and the zona pellucida prevents penetration by other spermatozoa.

The head of the spermatozoon then fuses with the ovum nucleus, creating a cell nucleus with 46 chromosomes. The fertilized ovum is called a *zygote*.

Pregnancy

Pregnancy starts with fertilization and ends with childbirth; on average, its duration is 38 weeks. During this period (called *gestation*), the zygote divides as it passes through the fallopian tube and attaches to the uterine lining via implantation. A complex sequence of *pre-embryonic*, *embryonic*, and *fetal* development transforms the zygote into a full-term fetus.

Making predictions

Because the uterus grows throughout pregnancy, uterine size serves as a rough estimate of gestation. The fertilization date is rarely known, so the woman's expected delivery date is typically calculated from the beginning of her last menses. The tool used for calculating delivery dates is known as *Nägele's rule.*

Here's how it works: If you know the first day of the last menstrual cycle, simply count back 3 months from that date and then add 7 days. For example, let's say that the first day of the last menses was April 29. Count back 3 months, which gets you to January 29, and then add 7 days for an approximate due date of February 5.

Stages of fetal development

During pregnancy, the fetus undergoes three major stages of development:

- pre-embryonic period
- embryonic period
- fetal period.

Rite of passage

The preembryonic phase starts with ovum fertilization and lasts for 2 weeks. As the zygote passes through the fallopian tube, it undergoes a series of *mitotic divisions*, or *cleavage*. (See *Pre-embryonic development*.)

Now I get it!

Pre-embryonic development

The pre-embryonic phase lasts from conception until approximately the end of the second week of development.

Zygote formation…

As the fertilized ovum advances through the fallopian tube toward the uterus, it undergoes mitotic division, forming daughter cells, initially called *blastomeres,* that each contain the same number of chromosomes as the parent cell. The first cell division ends about 30 hours after fertilization; subsequent divisions occur rapidly.

The *zygote,* as it's now called, develops into a small mass of cells called a *morula,* which reaches the uterus at or around the 3rd day after fertilization. Fluid that amasses in the center of the morula forms a central cavity.

…into blastocyst

The structure is now called a *blastocyst.* The blastocyst consists of a thin trophoblast layer, which includes the blastocyst cavity, and the inner cell mass. The trophoblast develops into fetal membranes and the placenta. The inner cell mass later forms the embryo *(late blastocyst).*

Getting attached: Blastocyst and endometrium

During the next phase, the blastocyst stays within the zona pellucida, unattached to the uterus. The zona pellucida degenerates and, by the end of the 1st week after fertilization, the blastocyst attaches to the endometrium. The part of the blastocyst adjacent to the inner cell mass is the first part to become attached.

The trophoblast, in contact with the endometrial lining, proliferates and invades the underlying endometrium by separating and dissolving endometrial cells.

Letting it all sink in

During the next week, the invading blastocyst sinks below the endometrium's surface. The penetration site seals, restoring the continuity of the endometrial surface.

Now I get it!

Embryonic development

Each of the three germ layers—ectoderm, mesoderm, and endoderm—forms specific tissues and organs in the developing embryo.

Ectoderm
The ectoderm, the outermost layer, develops into the:
• epidermis
• nervous system
• pituitary gland
• tooth enamel
• salivary glands
• optic lens
• lining of the lower portion of the anal canal
• hair.

Mesoderm
The mesoderm, the middle layer, develops into:
• connective and supporting tissue
• the blood and vascular system
• musculature
• teeth (except enamel)
• the mesothelial lining of the pericardial, pleural, and peritoneal cavities
• the kidneys and ureters.

Endoderm
The endoderm, the innermost layer, becomes the epithelial lining of the:
• pharynx and trachea
• auditory canal
• alimentary canal
• liver
• pancreas
• bladder and urethra
• prostate.

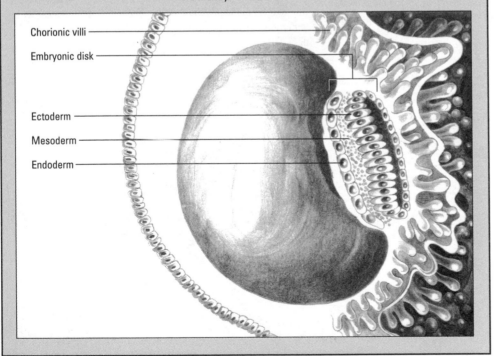

Chorionic villi
Embryonic disk
Ectoderm
Mesoderm
Endoderm

Look, honey — it has your germ layers...

During the embryonic period (gestation weeks 3 through 8), the developing zygote starts to take on a human shape and is now called an *embryo*. Each germ layer — the *ectoderm, mesoderm,* and *endoderm* — eventually forms specific tissues in the embryo. (See *Embryonic development.*)

...my organ systems...

The organ systems form during the embryonic period. During this time, the embryo is particularly vulnerable to injury by maternal drug use, certain maternal infections, and other factors.

...and a very large head

During the *fetal* stage of development, which lasts from the 9th week until birth, the maturing fetus enlarges and grows heavier. (See *From embryo to fetus*, page 296.)

Two unusual features appear during this stage:

The fetus's head is disproportionately large compared with its body. (This feature changes after birth as the infant grows.)

The fetus lacks subcutaneous fat. (Fat starts to accumulate shortly after birth.)

Memory jogger

To remember the three germ layers, keep in mind that *ecto* means outside, *meso* means middle, and *endo* means within.

Structural changes in the ovaries and uterus

Pregnancy changes the usual development of the *corpus luteum* (the ovum after ovulation, which secretes progesterone and small amounts of estrogen) and results in development of the decidua, amniotic sac and fluid, yolk sac, and placenta.

Corpus luteum

Normal functioning of the corpus luteum requires continual stimulation by *luteinizing hormone (LH)*. Progesterone produced by the corpus luteum suppresses LH release by the pituitary gland. If pregnancy occurs, the corpus luteum continues to produce progesterone until the placenta takes over. Otherwise, the corpus luteum atrophies 3 days before menstrual flow begins.

The fetus isn't the only thing changing during pregnancy — the reproductive system undergoes changes as well.

Now I get it!

From embryo to fetus

Significant growth and development take place within the first 3 months following conception, as the embryo develops into a fetus that nearly resembles a full-term newborn.

Month 1

At the end of the first month, the embryo has a definite form. The head, the trunk, and the tiny buds that will become the arms and legs are discernible. The cardiovascular system has begun to function, and the umbilical cord is visible in its most primitive form.

Month 2

During the second month, the embryo — called a *fetus* from the ninth week — grows to 1" (2.5 cm) in length and weighs ⅓₀ oz (1 g). The head and facial features develop as the eyes, ears, nose, lips, tongue, and tooth buds form. The arms and legs also take shape. Although the gender of the fetus isn't yet discernible, all external genitalia are present. Cardiovascular function is complete, and the umbilical cord has a definite form. At the end of the second month, the fetus resembles a full-term newborn, except for size.

Month 3

During the third month, the fetus grows to 3" (7.5 cm) in length and weighs 1 oz (28 g). Teeth and bones begin to appear, and the kidneys start to function. The fetus opens its mouth to swallow, grasps with its fully developed hands, and prepares for breathing by inhaling and exhaling amniotic fluid (although its lungs aren't functioning). At the end of the first *trimester* (the 3-month periods into which pregnancy is divided), the fetus's gender is distinguishable.

Months 4 to 9

Over the remaining 6 months, fetal growth continues as internal and external structures develop at a rapid rate. In the third trimester, the fetus stores the fats and minerals it will need to live outside the womb. At birth, the average full-term fetus measures 20" (51 cm) and weighs 7 to 7½ lb (3 to 3.5 kg).

1 month   2 months   3 months   9 months

Hormone soup

With age, the corpus luteum grows less responsive to LH. For this reason, the mature corpus luteum degenerates unless stimulated by progressively increasing amounts of LH.

Pregnancy stimulates the placental tissue to secrete large amounts of human chorionic gonadotropin (HCG), which resembles LH and follicle-stimulating hormone (FSH), also produced by the pituitary gland. HCG prevents corpus luteum degeneration, stimulating the corpus luteum to produce large amounts of estrogen and progesterone.

HCG tells all

The corpus luteum, stimulated by the hormone HCG, produces the estrogen and progesterone needed to maintain the pregnancy during the first 3 months. HCG can be detected as early as 9 days after fertilization and can provide confirmation of pregnancy even before the woman has missed her first menstrual period.

The HCG level gradually increases during this time, peaks at about 10 weeks' gestation, and then gradually declines.

Decidua

The *decidua* is the endometrial lining that undergoes the hormone-induced changes of pregnancy. Decidual cells secrete the following three substances:
• the hormone *prolactin*, which promotes lactation
• a peptide hormone, *relaxin*, which induces relaxation of the connective tissue of the symphysis pubis and pelvic ligaments and promotes cervical dilation
• a potent hormonelike fatty acid, *prostaglandin*, which mediates several physiologic functions.

(See *Development of the decidua and fetal membranes*, page 298.)

Amniotic sac and fluid

The *amniotic sac*, enclosed within the chorion, gradually enlarges and surrounds the embryo. As it grows, the amniotic sac expands into the chorionic cavity, eventually filling the cavity and fusing with the chorion by 8 weeks' gestation.

Development of the decidua and fetal membranes

Specialized tissues support, protect, and nurture the embryo and fetus throughout its development. Among these tissues, the decidua and fetal membranes begin to develop shortly after conception.

Nesting place

During pregnancy, the endometrial lining is called the *decidua*. It provides a nesting place for the developing ovum and has some endocrine functions.

Based primarily on its position relative to the embryo (see below), the decidua may be known as the *decidua basalis,* which lies beneath the *chorionic vesicle,* the *decidua capsularis,* which stretches over the vesicle, or the *decidua parietalis,* which lines the rest of the endometrial cavity.

Network of blood vessels

The *chorion* is a membrane that forms the outer wall of the blastocyst. Vascular projections, called *chorionic villi,* arise from its periphery. As the *chorionic vesicle* enlarges, villi arising from the superficial portion of the chorion, called the *chorion laeve,* atrophy, leaving this surface smooth. Villi arising from the deeper part of the chorion, called the *chorion frondosum,* proliferate, projecting into the large blood vessels within the decidua basalis through which the maternal blood flows.

Blood vessels form within the villi as they grow and connect with blood vessels that form in the chorion, in the body stalk, and within the body of the embryo. Blood begins to flow through this developing network of vessels as soon as the embryo's heart starts to beat.

Approximately 4 weeks

Decidua basalis
Chorionic vesicle
Amnion
Yolk sac
Decidua parietalis
Decidua capsularis
Cervix
Vagina

Approximately 16 weeks

Chorion frondosum
Decidua basalis
Yolk sac
Amnion
Chorion laeve

A warm, protective sea

The amniotic sac and amniotic fluid serve the fetus in two important ways—one during gestation and the other during delivery. During gestation, the fluid provides the fetus with a buoyant, temperature-controlled environment. Later, it serves as a fluid wedge that helps open the cervix during birth.

This is the life—warm, buoyant, and protected!

Thanks, mom — I'll take it from here

Early in pregnancy, amniotic fluid comes chiefly from three sources:

🖐 fluid filtering into the amniotic sac from maternal blood as it passes through the uterus

🖐 fluid filtering into the sac from fetal blood passing through the placenta

🖐 fluid diffusing into the amniotic sac from the fetal skin and respiratory tract.

Later in pregnancy, when the fetal kidneys begin to function, the fetus urinates into the amniotic fluid. Fetal urine then becomes the major source of amniotic fluid.

Daily gulps

Production of amniotic fluid from maternal and fetal sources compensates for amniotic fluid that's lost through the fetal GI tract. Normally, the fetus swallows up to several hundred milliliters of amniotic fluid each day. The fluid is absorbed into the fetal circulation from the fetal GI tract; some is transferred from the fetal circulation to the maternal circulation and excreted in maternal urine.

Yolk sac

The *yolk sac* forms next to the endoderm; a portion of it is incorporated in the developing embryo and forms the GI tract. Another portion of the sac develops into primitive germ cells, which travel to the developing gonads and eventually form *oocytes* (precursors to ova) or *spermatocytes* (precursors to spermatozoa), after gender is determined at fertilization.

No yolk — it's only temporary

During early embryonic development, the yolk sac also forms blood cells. Eventually, it atrophies and disintegrates.

Placenta

The flattened, disk-shaped *placenta,* using the umbilical cord as its conduit, provides nutrients to and removes wastes from the fetus from the third month of pregnancy until birth. The placenta is formed from the chorion, its chorionic villi, and the adjacent decidua basalis.

The strongest link

The umbilical cord, which contains two arteries and one vein, links the fetus to the placenta. The umbilical arteries, which transport blood from the fetus to the placenta, take a spiral course on the cord, divide on the placental surface, and branch off to the chorionic villi. (See *Picturing the placenta.*)

In a helpful vein

The placenta is a highly vascular organ. Large veins on its surface gather blood returning from the villi and join to form the single umbilical vein. The umbilical vein enters the cord, returning blood to the fetus.

Specialists on the job

The placenta contains two highly specialized circulatory systems:
• The *uteroplacental* circulation carries oxygenated arterial blood from the maternal circulation to the *intervillous spaces* — large spaces separating chorionic villi in the placenta. Blood enters the intervillous spaces from uterine arteries that penetrate the basal portion of the placenta; it leaves the intervillous spaces and flows back into the maternal circulation through veins in the basal portion of the placenta near the arteries.
• The *fetoplacental* circulation transports oxygen-depleted blood from the fetus to the chorionic villi through the umbilical arteries and returns oxygenated blood to the fetus through the umbilical vein.

Zoom in

Picturing the placenta

At term, the *placenta* (the spongy structure within the uterus from which the fetus derives nourishment) is flat, pancakelike, and round or oval. It measures 6″ to 7¾″ (15 to 20 cm) in diameter and ¾″ to 1¼″ (2 to 3 cm) in breadth at its thickest part. The maternal side is lobulated; the fetal side is shiny.

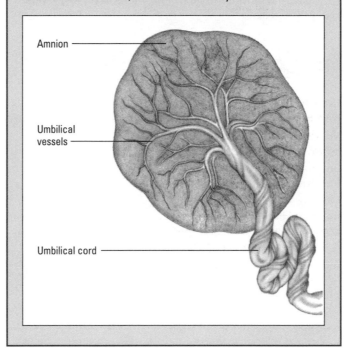

Amnion

Umbilical vessels

Umbilical cord

Placenta takes charge

For the first 3 months of pregnancy, the corpus luteum is the main source of estrogen and progesterone — steroid hormones required during pregnancy. By the end of the third month, however, the placenta produces most of the hormones; the corpus luteum persists but is no longer needed to maintain the pregnancy.

Hormones on the rise

Levels of estrogen and progesterone increase progressively throughout pregnancy. Estrogen stimulates uterine development to provide a suitable environment for the fetus. Progesterone, synthesized by the placenta from maternal cholesterol, reduces uterine muscle irritability and prevents spontaneous abortion of the fetus.

Keep those acids coming

The placenta also produces *human placental lactogen* (HPL), which resembles growth hormone. HPL stimulates maternal protein and fat metabolism to ensure a sufficient supply of amino acids and fatty acids for the mother and fetus. HPL also stimulates breast growth in preparation for lactation. Throughout pregnancy, HPL levels rise progressively.

Labor and the postpartum period

Childbirth is achieved through labor — the process by which uterine contractions expel the fetus from the uterus. When labor begins, these contractions become strong and regular. Eventually, voluntary bearing-down efforts supplement the contractions, resulting in delivery. When that occurs, presentation of the fetus takes one of a variety of forms. (See *Comparing fetal presentations.*)

Get ready to work! The contractions of labor are involuntary at first but are supplemented by voluntary efforts as birth approaches.

Onset of labor

The onset of labor results from several factors:
• The number of *oxytocin* (a pituitary hormone that stimulates uterine contractions) receptors on uterine muscle fibers increases progressively during pregnancy, peaking just before labor onset. This makes the uterus more sensitive to the effects of oxytocin.
• Stretching of the uterus over the course of the pregnancy initiates nerve impulses that stimulate oxytocin secretion from the posterior pituitary lobe.

Now I get it!

Comparing fetal presentations

Fetal presentations may be broadly classified as cephalic, breech, shoulder, or compound.

Cephalic
In the *cephalic*, or head-down presentation, the position of the fetus may be classified further by the presenting skull landmark, such as vertex (the topmost part of the head), brow, sinciput (the forward, upper part of the skull), or face.

Breech
In the *breech,* or head-up, presentation, the position of the fetus may be further classified as frank (hip flexed, knees straight), complete (knees and hips flexed), footling (knees and hips of one or both legs extended), kneeling (knees flexed and hips extended), or incomplete (one or both hips extended and one or both feet or knees lying below the breech).

Shoulder
Although a fetus may adopt one of several *shoulder* presentations, examination won't help a practitioner differentiate among them. Thus, all transverse positions are called *shoulder presentations.*

Compound
In a *compound* presentation, an extremity prolapses alongside the major presenting part so that two presenting parts appear at the pelvis at the same time.

Cephalic	Complete breech	Shoulder	Compound

Initiating start sequence

Near term, the fetal pituitary gland secretes more *adreno-corticotropic* hormone, which causes the fetal adrenal glands to secrete more *cortisol*. The cortisol diffuses into the maternal circulation through the placenta, heightens oxytocin and estrogen secretion, and reduces progesterone secretion. These changes intensify uterine muscle irritability and make the uterus even more sensitive to oxytocin stimulation.

Decline, diffuse, and contract

Declining progesterone levels convert *esterified arachidonic acid* into a nonesterified form. The nonesterified arachidonic acid undergoes biosynthesis to form prostaglandins which, in turn, diffuse into the *uterine myometrium*, thereby inducing uterine contractions.

All systems go

As the cervix dilates, nerve impulses are transmitted to the central nervous system, causing an increase in oxytocin secretion from the pituitary gland. Acting as a positive feedback mechanism, increased oxytocin secretion stimulates more uterine contractions, which further dilate the cervix and lead the pituitary to secrete more oxytocin. Oxytocin secretions may also stimulate *prostaglandin* formation by the decidua.

Stages of labor

Childbirth can be divided into three stages. The duration of each stage varies according to the size of the uterus, the woman's age, and the number of previous pregnancies.

Stage 1 — efface and dilate

The first stage of labor, in which the fetus begins its descent, is marked by cervical *effacement* (thinning) and *dilation*. Before labor begins, the cervix isn't dilated; by the end of the first stage, it has dilated fully. The first stage of labor can last from 6 to 24 hours in primiparous women but is commonly significantly shorter for multiparous women. (See *Cervical effacement and dilation.*)

Cervical effacement and dilation

Cervical effacement and dilation are significant aspects of the first stage of labor.

Thinning walls

Cervical effacement is the progressive shortening of the vaginal portion of the cervix and the thinning of its walls during labor as it's stretched by the fetus. Effacement is described as a percentage, ranging from 0% (non-effaced and thick) to 100% (fully effaced and paper-thin).

Bigger exit

Cervical dilation refers to progressive enlargement of the *cervical os* to allow the fetus to pass from the uterus into the vagina. Dilation ranges from less than 1 cm to about 10 cm (full dilation).

No effacement or dilation

Internal os
Cavity of cervix
External os

Early effacement and dilation

Internal os
External os

Complete effacement and dilation

Internal os

External os

Stage 2 — no turning back

The second stage of labor begins with full cervical dilation and ends with delivery of the fetus. During this stage, the amniotic sac ruptures as the uterine contractions increase in frequency and intensity. (The amniotic sac can also rupture before the onset of labor — during the first stage — and, although rare, sometimes ruptures after expulsion of the fetus.) As the flexed head of the fetus enters the pelvis, the mother's pelvic muscles force the head to rotate anteriorly and cause the back of the head to move under the symphysis pubis.

The first stage of labor can last from 6 to 24 hours in primiparous women; the second stage lasts only about 45 minutes.

The curtain rises

As the uterus contracts, the flexed head of the fetus is forced deeper into the pelvis; resistance of the pelvic floor gradually forces the head to extend. As the head presses against the pelvic floor, vulvar tissues stretch and the anus dilates.

The star appears

The head of the fetus now rotates back to its former position after passing through the vulvovaginal orifice. Usually, head rotation is lateral (external) as the anterior shoulder rotates forward to pass under the pubic arch. Delivery of the shoulders and the rest of the fetus follows. The second stage of labor averages about 45 minutes in primiparous women; it may be much shorter in multiparous women.

Both stages are typically much shorter for women who have delivered before.

Curtain call

The third stage of labor starts immediately after childbirth and ends with placenta expulsion. After the neonate is delivered, the uterus continues to contract intermittently and grows smaller. The area of placental attachment also decreases. The placenta, which can't decrease in size, separates from the uterus, and blood seeps into the area of placental separation. The third stage of labor averages about 10 minutes in primiparous and multiparous women.

Postpartum period

After childbirth, the reproductive tract takes about 6 weeks to revert to its former condition during a process called *involution.* The uterus quickly grows smaller, with most of its involution taking place during the first 2 weeks after delivery.

Discharged with honors

Postpartum vaginal discharge (lochia) persists for several weeks after childbirth:
• *Lochia rubra,* a bloody discharge, occurs immediately after delivery and lasts for 1 to 4 days postpartum.
• *Lochia serosa,* a pinkish brown, serous discharge, occurs from 5 to 7 days postpartum.
• *Lochia alba,* a grayish white or colorless discharge, appears from 1 to 3 weeks postpartum.

Lactation

Lactation (milk synthesis and secretion by the breasts) is governed by interactions involving four hormones:
• estrogen and progesterone, produced by the ovaries and placenta
• prolactin and oxytocin, produced by the pituitary gland under hypothalamic control.

Hormonal initiation of lactation

As gestation progresses, the production of estrogen and progesterone by the placenta increases, causing glandular and ductal tissue in the breasts to proliferate. After breast stimulation by estrogen and progesterone, prolactin causes milk secretion.

Priming the pump

Oxytocin from the posterior pituitary lobe causes contraction of specialized cells in the breast, producing a squeezing effect that forces milk down the ducts. Breastfeeding, in turn, stimulates prolactin secretion, resulting in a high prolactin level that induces changes in the menstrual cycle.

Opening the throttle

Progesterone and estrogen levels fall after delivery. With estrogen and progesterone no longer inhibiting prolactin's effects on milk production, the mammary glands start to secrete milk.

Pressing on the gas pedal

Nipple stimulation during breast-feeding results in transmission of sensory impulses from the nipples to the hypothalamus. If the nipples aren't stimulated by breast-feeding, prolactin secretion declines after delivery. Milk secretion continues as long as breast-feeding regularly stimulates the nipples. If breast-feeding stops, the stimulus for prolactin release is eliminated and milk production ceases.

Regular breast-feeding provides the stimulus necessary for continued milk production.

Breast-feeding and the menstrual cycle

During the postpartum period, the woman's high prolactin level inhibits FSH and LH release. If she doesn't breast-feed, her prolactin output soon drops, ending inhibition of FSH and LH production by the pituitary. Subsequently, cyclic release of FSH and LH occurs. (See *Breast milk composition.*)

Breast milk composition

The composition of breast milk undergoes various changes during the process of lactation.

First tastes
Initial feedings provide a thin, serous fluid called colostrum. Unlike mature breast milk, which has a bluish tinge, colostrum is yellow. Colostrum contains high concentrations of protein, fat-soluble vitamins, minerals, and immunoglobulins, which function as antibodies. Its laxative effect promotes early passage of meconium, the greenish black material that collects in the fetal intestines and forms the neonate's first stool. The breasts may contain colostrum for up to 96 hours after delivery.

From foremilk to hindmilk
Breast milk composition continues to change over the course of a feeding. The foremilk — the thin, watery milk secreted when a feeding begins — is low in calories but abounds in water-soluble vitamins. It accounts for about 60% of the total volume of a feeding. Next, hindmilk is released. The hindmilk, available 10 to 15 minutes after a breast-feeding session begins, has the highest concentration of calories; this helps to satisfy the neonate's hunger between feedings.

A hold on ovulation

In a breast-feeding woman, the menstrual cycle doesn't resume because prolactin inhibits the cyclic release of FSH and LH necessary for ovulation. This explains why a breast-feeding woman usually doesn't become pregnant.

The cycle comes full circle

Prolactin release in response to breast-feeding gradually declines, as does the inhibitory effect of prolactin on FSH and LH release. Consequently, ovulation and the menstrual cycle may resume. Pregnancy may occur after this, even if the woman continues to breast-feed.

Quick quiz

1. Each of the three germ layers (ectoderm, mesoderm, and endoderm) forms specific tissues and organs in the developing:

    A. zygote.
    B. ovum.
    C. embryo.
    D. fetus.

Answer: C. Each of the three germ layers (ectoderm, mesoderm, and endoderm) forms specific tissues and organs in the developing embryo.

2. Which structure is responsible for protecting the fetus?

    A. Decidua
    B. Amniotic fluid
    C. Corpus luteum
    D. Yolk sac

Answer: B. Amniotic fluid, which provides a buoyant, temperature-controlled environment, protects the fetus.

3. Progressive enlargement of the cervical os during labor is called:

    A. dilation.
    B. effacement.
    C. lactation.
    D. differentiation.

Answer: A. The progressive enlargement of the cervical os during labor is called *dilation*.

4. The initial breast milk that's yellow in color is called:
   A. foremilk.
   B. hindmilk.
   C. colostrum.
   D. prolactin.

Answer: C. The initial breast milk that's yellow in color is called *colostrum*.

Scoring

☆☆☆ If you answered all four questions correctly, fabulous! You're first-rate with the physiology of fertilization.

☆☆ If you answered three questions correctly, excellent! You're looking good in the areas of labor and lactation.

☆ If you answered fewer than three questions correctly, don't be alarmed! Cycling through the information in the chapter again should guarantee you won't reproduce those results.

Appendices and index

Glossary

abdomen
area of the body between the diaphragm and pelvis

abduct
to move away from the midline of the body; the opposite of *adduct*

acetabulum
hip joint socket into which the head of the femur fits

acromion
bony projection of the scapula

adduct
to move toward the midline of the body; the opposite of *abduct*

adenoids
paired lymphoid structures located in the nasopharynx

adrenal gland
one of two secretory organs that lie atop the kidneys; consists of a medulla and a cortex

afferent neuron
nerve cell that conveys impulses from the periphery to the central nervous system; the opposite of *efferent neuron*

alveolus
small saclike dilation of the terminal bronchioles in the lung

ampulla
saclike dilation of a tube or duct

anterior
front or ventral; the opposite of *posterior* or *dorsal*

antibody
immunoglobulin produced by the body in response to exposure to a specific foreign substance (antigen)

antigen
foreign substance that causes antibody formation when introduced into the body

anus
distal end or outlet of the rectum

aorta
main trunk of the systemic arterial circulation, originating from the left ventricle and eventually branching into the two common iliac arteries

arachnoid
delicate middle membrane of the meninges

areola
pigmented ring around the nipple

arteriole
small branch of an artery

artery
vessel that carries blood away from the heart

arthrosis
joint or articulation

atrium
chamber or cavity

auricle
part of the ear that's attached to the head

axon
extension of a nerve cell that conveys impulses away from the cell body

bladder
membranous sac that holds secretions

bone
dense, hard connective tissue that composes the skeleton

bone marrow
soft tissue in the cancellous bone of the epiphyses; crucial for blood cell formation and maturation

bronchiole
small branch of the bronchus

bronchus
larger air passage of the lung

buccal
pertaining to the cheek

312

bursa
fluid-filled sac lined with synovial membrane

capillary
microscopic blood vessel that links arterioles with venules

carpal
pertaining to the wrist

cartilage
connective supporting tissue occurring mainly in the joints, thorax, larynx, trachea, nose, and ear

cecum
pouch located at the proximal end of the large intestine

celiac
pertaining to the abdomen

central nervous system
one of the two main divisions of the nervous system; consists of the brain and spinal cord

cerebellum
portion of the brain situated in the posterior cranial fossa, behind the brain stem; coordinates voluntary muscular activity

cerebrum
largest and uppermost section of the brain, divided into hemispheres

cilia
small, hairlike projections on the outer surfaces of some cells

cochlea
spiral tube that makes up a portion of the inner ear

colon
part of the large intestine that extends from the cecum to the rectum

condyle
rounded projection at the end of a bone

contralateral
on the opposite side; the opposite of *ipsilateral*

cornea
convex, transparent anterior portion of the eye

coronary
pertaining to the heart or its arteries

cortex
outer part of an internal organ; the opposite of *medulla*

costal
pertaining to the ribs

cricoid
ring-shaped cartilage found in the larynx

cutaneous
pertaining to the skin

deltoid
shaped like a triangle (as in the deltoid muscle)

dendrite
branching process extending from the neuronal cell body that directs impulses toward the cell body

dermis
skin layer beneath the epidermis

diaphragm
membrane that separates one part from another; the muscular partition separating the thorax and abdomen

diaphysis
shaft of a long bone

diarthrosis
freely movable joint

diencephalon
part of the brain located between the cerebral hemisphere and the midbrain

distal
far from the point of origin or attachment; the opposite of *proximal*

diverticulum
outpouching from a tubular organ such as the intestine

dorsal
pertaining to the back or posterior; the opposite of *ventral* or *anterior*

duct
passage or canal

duodenum
shortest and widest portion of the small intestine, extending from the pylorus to the jejunum

dura mater
outermost layer of the meninges

ear
organ of hearing

efferent neuron
nerve cell that conveys impulses from the central nervous system to the periphery; the opposite of *afferent neuron*

endocardium
interior lining of the heart

endocrine
pertaining to secretion into the blood or lymph rather than into a duct; the opposite of *exocrine*

epidermis
outermost layer of the skin; lacking vessels

epiglottis
cartilaginous structure overhanging the larynx that guards against entry of food into the lung

epiphyses
ends of a long bone

erythrocyte
red blood cell

esophagus
muscular canal that transports nutrients from the pharynx to the stomach

exocrine
pertaining to secretion into a duct; the opposite of *endocrine*

eye
one of two organs of vision

fallopian tube
one of two ducts extending from the uterus to the ovary

fontanel
incompletely ossified area of a neonate's skull

foramen
small opening

fossa
hollow or cavity

fundus
base of a hollow organ; the part farthest from the organ's outlet

gallbladder
excretory sac lodged in the visceral surface of the liver's right lobe

ganglion
cluster of nerve cell bodies found outside the central nervous system

genitalia
reproductive organs; may be external or internal

gland
organ or structure body that secretes or excretes substances

glomerulus
compact cluster; the capillaries of the kidney

gonad
sex gland in which reproductive cells form

heart
muscular, cone-shaped organ that pumps blood throughout the body

hemoglobin
protein found in red blood cells that contains iron

hormone
substance secreted by an endocrine gland that triggers or regulates the activity of an organ or cell group

hyoid
shaped like the letter U; the U-shaped bone at the base of the tongue

hypothalamus
structure in the diencephalon that secretes vasopressin and oxytocin

ileum
distal part of the small intestine extending from the jejunum to the cecum

incus
one of three bones in the middle ear

inferior
lower; the opposite of *superior*

intestine
portion of the GI tract that extends from the stomach to the anus

intima
innermost structure

ipsilateral
on the same side; the opposite of *contralateral*

jejunum
one of three portions of the small intestine; connects proximally with the duodenum and distally with the ileum

joint
fibrous, cartilaginous, or synovial connection between bones

kidney
one of two urinary organs on the dorsal part of the abdomen

labia
lips

lacrimal
pertaining to tears

larynx
voice organ; joins the pharynx and trachea

lateral
pertaining to the side; the opposite of *medial*

leukocyte
white blood cell

ligament
band of white fibrous tissue that connects bones

liver
large gland in the right upper abdomen; divided into four lobes

lobe
defined portion of any organ, such as the liver or brain

lobule
small lobe

lumbar
pertaining to the area of the back between the thorax and the pelvis

lungs
organs of respiration found in the chest's lateral cavities

lymph
watery fluid in lymphatic vessels

lymph node
small oval structure that filters lymph, fights infection, and aids hematopoiesis

lymphocyte
white blood cell; the body's immunologically competent cells

malleolus
projections at the distal ends of the tibia and fibula

malleus
tiny hammer-shaped bone in the middle ear

mammary
pertaining to the breast

manubrium
upper part of the sternum

meatus
opening or passageway

medial
pertaining to the middle; the opposite of *lateral*

mediastinum
middle portion of the thorax between the pleural sacs that contain the lungs

medulla
inner portion of an organ; the opposite of *cortex*

membrane
thin layer or sheet

metacarpals
bones of the hand located between the wrist and the fingers

metatarsals
bones of the foot located between the tarsal bones and the toes

muscle
fibrous structure whose contraction initiates movement

myocardium
thick, contractile layer of muscle cells that forms the heart wall

nares
nostrils

nephron
structural and functional unit of the kidney

nerve
cordlike structure consisting of fibers that convey impulses from the central nervous system to the body

neuron
nerve cell

neutrophil
white blood cell that removes and destroys bacteria, cellular debris, and solid particles

occiput
back of the head

olfactory
pertaining to the sense of smell

ophthalmic
pertaining to the eye

ossicle
small bone, especially of the ear

ovary
one of two female reproductive organs found on each side of the lower abdomen, next to the uterus

palate
roof of the mouth

pancreas
secretory gland in the epigastric and hypogastric regions

parotid
located near the ear (as in the parotid gland)

patella
floating bone that forms the kneecap

pectoral
pertaining to the chest or breast

pelvis
funnel-shaped structure; lower part of the trunk

pericardium
fibroserous sac that surrounds the heart and the origin of the great vessels

phalanx
one of the tapering bones that makes up the fingers and toes

pharynx
tubular passageway that extends from the base of the skull to the esophagus

phrenic
pertaining to the diaphragm

pia mater
innermost covering of the brain and spinal cord

pituitary gland
gland attached to the hypothalamus that stores and secretes hormones

plantar
pertaining to the sole of the foot

plasma
colorless, watery fluid portion of lymph and blood

platelet
small, disk-shaped blood cell necessary for coagulation

pleura
thin serous membrane that encloses the lung

plexus
network of nerves, lymphatic vessels, or veins

pons
portion of the brain that lies between the medulla and the mesencephalon

popliteal
pertaining to the back of the knee

posterior
back or dorsal; the opposite of *anterior* or *ventral*

pronate
to turn the palm downward; the opposite of *supinate*

prostate
male gland that surrounds the bladder neck and urethra

proximal
situated nearest the center of the body; the opposite of *distal*

pupil
circular opening in the iris of the eye through which light passes

reflex
involuntary action

renal
pertaining to the kidney

scrotum
skin pouch that houses the testes and parts of the spermatic cords

semen
male reproductive fluid

sphenoid
wedged-shaped bone at the base of the skull

spleen
highly vascular organ between the stomach and diaphragm

stapes
tiny stirrup-shaped bone in the middle ear

sternum
long, flat bone that forms the middle portion of the thorax

stomach
major digestive organ, located in the right upper abdomen

striated
marked with parallel lines such as striated (skeletal) muscle

superior
higher; the opposite of *inferior*

supinate
to turn the palm of the hand upward; the opposite of *pronate*

symphysis
growing together; a type of cartilaginous joint in which fibrocartilage firmly connects opposing surfaces

synapse
point of contact between adjacent neurons

systole
contraction of the heart muscle

talus
anklebone

tarsus
instep

tendon
band of fibrous connective tissue that attaches a muscle to a bone

testis
one of two male gonads that produce semen

thyroid
secretory gland located at the front of the neck

tibia
shinbone

tongue
chief organ of taste, found in the floor of the mouth

trachea
nearly cylindrical tube in the neck, extending from the larynx to the bronchi, that serves as a passageway for air

turbinate
shaped like a cone or spiral; a bone located in the posterior nasopharynx

ureter
one of two thick-walled tubes that transport urine to the bladder

urethra
small tubular structure that drains urine from the bladder

uterus
hollow, internal female reproductive organ in which the fertilized ovum is implanted and the fetus develops

uvula
tissue projection that hangs from the soft palate

vagina
sheath; the canal in the female extending from the vulva to the cervix

valve
structure that permits fluid to flow in only one direction

vein
vessel that carries blood to the heart

vena cava
one of two large veins that returns blood from the peripheral circulation to the right atrium

ventral
pertaining to the front or anterior; the opposite of *dorsal* or *posterior*

ventricle
small cavity, such as one of several in the brain or one of the two lower chambers of the heart

venule
small vessel that connects a vein and capillary plexuses

vertebra
any of the 33 bones that make up the spinal column

viscera
internal organs

xiphoid
sword-shaped; the lower portion of the sternum

Selected references

Atlas of Human Anatomy. Springhouse, Pa.: Lippincott Williams & Wilkins, 2001.

Atlas of Pathophysiology. Springhouse, Pa.: Lippincott Williams & Wilkins, 2002.

Baggaley, A. *Human Body: An Illustrated Guide to Every Part of the Human Body and How It Works.* New York: Dorling Kindersley Publishing, Inc., 2001.

Gavaghan, M. "The Pancreas — Hermit of the Abdomen," *AORN Journal* 75(6):1110-4, 1117, 1119, June 2002.

Kindlen, S. *Physiology for Health Care and Nursing,* 2nd ed. London: Churchill Livingstone, 2003.

Lea, D.H. "Ahead to the Past: How Genetics Is Changing Your Practice," *Nursing2002* 32(6):48-51, June 2002.

Lippincott Professional Guides: Anatomy & Physiology, 2nd ed. Springhouse, Pa.: Lippincott Williams & Wilkins, 2002.

Nutrition Made Incredibly Easy! Springhouse, Pa.: Lippincott Williams & Wilkins, 2003.

Porth, C.M. *Essentials of Pathophysiology: Concepts of Altered Health States.* Philadelphia: Lippincott Williams & Wilkins, 2003.

Professional Guide to Pathophysiology. Springhouse, Pa.: Lippincott Williams & Wilkins, 2003.

Rohen, J.W., et al. *Color Atlas of Anatomy: A Photographic Study of the Human Body,* 5th ed. Philadelphia: Lippincott Williams & Wilkins, 2002.

Sheahan, S.L., and Musialowski, R. "Clinical Implications of Respiratory System Changes in Aging," *Journal of Gerontological Nursing* 27(5):26-34, May 2001.

Thibodeau, G.A., and Patton, K.T. *Anatomy and Physiology,* 5th ed. St. Louis: Mosby Year–Book, Inc., 2003.

Twietmeyer, A., and McCracken, T. *Coloring Guide to Human Anatomy,* 3rd ed. Philadelphia: Lippincott Williams & Wilkins, 2001.

Index

i refers to an illustration; t refers to a table; **boldface** refers to a full-color illustration.

i refers to an illustration; t refers to a table; **boldface** refers to a full-color illustration.

i refers to an illustration; t refers to a table; **boldface** refers to a full-color illustration.

i refers to an illustration; t refers to a table; **boldface** refers to a full-color illustration.